THE CARDIAC ARRHYTHMIAS

THE CARDIAC ARRHYTHMIAS

BRENDAN PHIBBS, M.D., F.A.C.P., F.A.C.C.

Associate Professor of Medicine, University of Arizona College of Medicine;
Director, Electrocardiographic Laboratory,
University Hospital, Tucson, Arizona

With contribution by

Gordon A. Ewy, M.D., F.A.C.C.

Associate Professor of Medicine, University of Arizona College of Medicine;
Director, Physiological Testing Laboratory and Coronary Care Unit,
University Hospital, Tucson, Arizona

SECOND EDITION

with 264 illustrations

THE C. V. MOSBY COMPANY

SAINT LOUIS   1973

SECOND EDITION

Copyright © 1973 by The C. V. Mosby Company

All rights reserved. No part of this book may be reproduced
in any manner without written permission of the publisher.

Printed in the United States of America

Previous edition copyrighted 1961

Distributed in Great Britain by Henry Kimpton, London

Library of Congress Cataloging in Publication Data

Phibbs, Brendan.
    The cardiac arrhythmias.

    1. Arrhythmia. I. Title.
[DNLM: 1. Arrhythmia. WG 330 P543c 1973]
RC685.A65P45 1973   616.1'28   73-4661
ISBN 0-8016-3910-7

VH/M/M 9 8 7 6 5 4 3

PREFACE

It was Sheridan who said, "Easy writing's curst hard reading." This book is an exercise on the other face of that coin: if the book has a virtue, it is simplicity. A lifetime of digging through jumbled syntax to unearth simple medical facts has convinced me that most scientific writing is needlessly obscure. Most scientific phenomena can be described in simple, clear, almost basic English, if the writer will take the trouble to do so. Most writers don't.

Don't be surprised, therefore, when you sometimes read that a pacemaker "fires" instead of "discharging," or when "anterograde propagation of the depolarizing impulse" is translated as "the wave moves down." This is deliberate. (As long as the term "wave" and the direction "down" are defined, the last two statements are identical.)

Bundle of His recordings are mentioned briefly; such recordings are of great research and theoretical interest and have illuminated many problems of conduction, but it is only in rare cases that the method yields practical clinical information. With a few exceptions, the necessary therapeutic and prognostic conclusions can be derived from the surface electrocardiogram.

Beta-adrenergic blocking agents are also mentioned sparingly. These drugs have been a boon in treatment of angina pectoris, but their usefulness in treating arrhythmias is limited by their unique toxicity. Better and safer agents that will control almost any cardiac arrhythmia are available; recurrent paroxysmal tachycardias in the young and tachyarrhythmias associated with preexcitation probably represent the only genuine indications for beta-blockade treatment of arrhythmias. Overenthusiastic use of this dangerous class of drug has certainly caused deaths from intractable heart failure: *primum nolle nocere!*

Finally, this is a basic book for the noncardiologist. For those who find the subject congenial, I would recommend the classic texts by Katz, Pick, and Langendorf and the current text by Chung, as well as the extensive and always excellent writings of Marriott and Schamroth, as entrees to the more recondite aspects of the cardiac arrhythmias.

Brendan Phibbs

CONTENTS

Part I BASIC ANATOMY AND PHYSIOLOGY

1 Anatomy and physiology of the conducting tissues of the heart, 3

2 Basic facts and measurements in the electrocardiogram, 8

Part II SIMPLE ARRHYTHMIAS

3 The sinus rhythms, 13

4 Ectopic beats, 16

5 Sustained ectopic rhythms, 29

6 Ventricular aberration and ventricular fusion, 44

7 Problems, practice, and reinforcement: 1, 50

8 Atrioventricular block, 59

9 Atrial fibrillation, 82

10 Atrial flutter, 91

11 Problems, practice, and reinforcement: 2, 98

Part III COMPLEX ARRHYTHMIAS

12 Digitalis-induced arrhythmias, 113

13 Interference, dissociation, and confusion, 128

14 Sick sinus syndrome, 135

15 Some complex arrhythmias, 142

16 Fatal arrhythmias; arrhythmias in the coronary care unit, 150

17 Wandering pacemaker; pre-excitation; criteria of aberration; parasystole, 158

18 Problems, practice, and reinforcement: 3, 164

Part IV DRUGS AND TECHNIQUE

19 Drugs and dosages, 179

20 Pacers and pacing, 185

21 Defibrillators, defibrillation, and cardioversion, 188

Part I
BASIC ANATOMY AND PHYSIOLOGY

1 Anatomy and physiology of the conducting tissues of the heart

ANATOMY

The essential anatomy of the conducting system of the heart is surprisingly simple: it consists of only six major parts (Fig. 1-1).

Sinoatrial (S-A) node. The S-A node is a small structure located in the right atrium near its junction with the superior vena cava. It is composed of a mass of specialized cells richly supplied with blood vessels.

Atrial syncytium. The atrial syncytium is the network of cells that forms the walls of the atria.

Atrioventricular (A-V) node. The A-V node is the structure lying in the upper portion of the interventricular septum near the entrance of the coronary sinus into the right atrium. It is composed of Purkinje fibers.

Bundle of His (atrioventricular bundle). The bundle of His is a continuation of the A-V node into the interventricular septum. The ultrastructure of the bundle of His, as seen in the electron microscope, is quite different from the structure of the A-V node.

RIGHT AND LEFT BRANCHES OF THE BUNDLE OF HIS. The common bundle quickly divides into two bundle branches, one going down each side of the interventricular septum.

Purkinje fibers. The Purkinje fibers are scattered throughout the subendocardium of the ventricles and represent the last link in the chain of excitation.

PHYSIOLOGY OF THE NORMAL HEARTBEAT (Fig. 1-2)

The S-A node is the normal pacemaker of the heart. It sends out an electric wave that traverses the conducting tissues of the heart, producing the muscular contraction of the heartbeat. Think of the atria as a large pond. Seated at one corner of the pond, you play the role of the S-A node. You do this by dropping a rock in the pond every second: each time, a ripple spreads evenly through the water.

There is a small outlet canal from the pond that soon divides into two main branches and then into a myriad of tiny channels. You note that part of the ripple you produce travels down the outlet canal and through all the channels to their extremities. This is a good representation of the spread of the exciting impulse through the heart.

It was formerly thought that the exciting wave started by the S-A node spread uniformly throughout the atrial tissues. Newer studies suggest that there are spe-

3

cialized pathways of conduction from the S-A node to the A-V node. While this information is of intense theoretical interest, it has no practical significance at this time.

A part of this wave front travels down the A-V node, into the bundle of His, out the two bundle branches, and through the network of nerve fibers in the ventricles.

A restoring or repolarizing wave travels back across the heart in the same fashion.

Correlation with waves of electrocardiogram

Fig. 1-2 shows the relation of these events to the deflections of the electrocardiogram (ECG). To diagnose arrhythmias by means of the electrocardiogram, one must be ready to use three sets of facts:

1. The P wave represents activation of the atria. The beginning of the upstroke of the P wave indicates the time atrial activation starts; the return of the P wave to

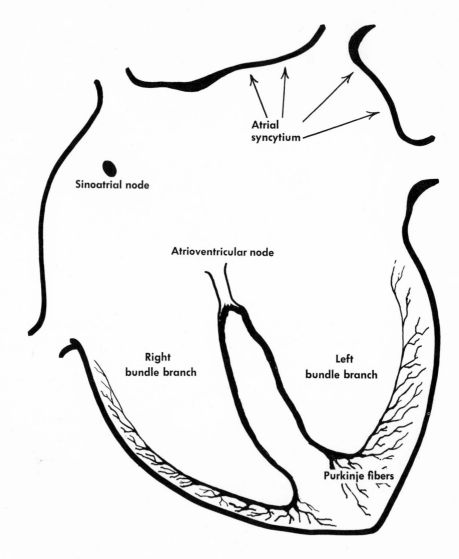

Fig. 1-1. Schematic representation of the conducting tissues of the heart.

the baseline indicates time of completion of atrial activation. In other words, the presence of a P wave indicates that atrial activation has taken place, and the width of the P wave tells the time required for completion of that activation.

2. No electric activity is recorded at the surface of the body during passage of the activating wave through the A-V node and bundle of His. The flat segment of the electrocardiogram from the end of the P wave to the beginning of the QRS indicates this "silent" passage.

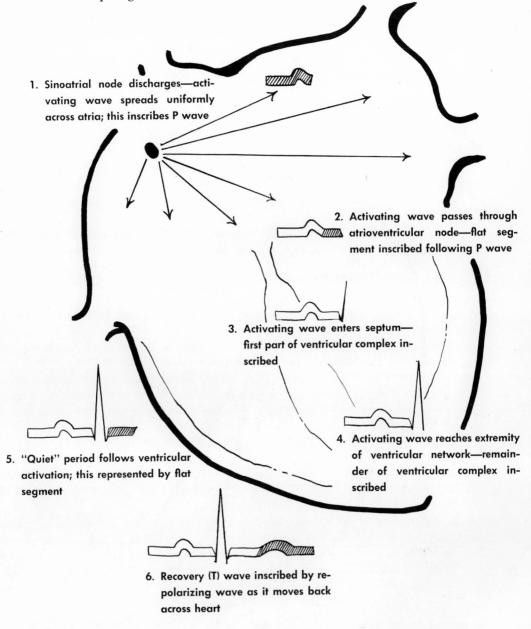

1. Sinoatrial node discharges—activating wave spreads uniformly across atria; this inscribes P wave

2. Activating wave passes through atrioventricular node—flat segment inscribed following P wave

3. Activating wave enters septum—first part of ventricular complex inscribed

4. Activating wave reaches extremity of ventricular network—remainder of ventricular complex inscribed

5. "Quiet" period follows ventricular activation; this represented by flat segment

6. Recovery (T) wave inscribed by repolarizing wave as it moves back across heart

Fig. 1-2. Sequence of events in electrical activation of the heart as registered on the electrocardiogram.

3. The ventricular conducting system begins at the "fork in the road" where the first branch of the bundle branch system leaves the common bundle of His. Inscription of the ventricular complex, or QRS complex, begins when the activating wave breaks out of the slowly conducting bundle of His and begins its swift course through the bundle branches. The QRS ends with the activation of the most remote part of the Purkinje network—the area around the crista supraventricularis in the right ventricle.

The presence of a ventricular complex indicates activation of the ventricular conducting system; the width of the ventricular complex tells how long that process takes.

EMPHASIS: Movement of an activating wave across any part of the atria or ventricles will always produce a deflection in the electrocardiogram, whether the chambers are activated in whole or in part. Movement of an activating wave through the A-V node and bundle of His is always silent, and the time required for such movement is indicated by the duration of a flat or isoelectric segment of the electrocardiogram, starting with the end of the P wave and ending with the beginning of the ventricular complex (in the case of normal activation).

Basic physiology facts

Nervous control of the conducting system. Both the sympathetic and the parasympathetic nerve fibers reach and influence the conducting tissues of the heart. They are basically completely opposite in their effects. Three sets of facts must be learned first:

1. Sympathetic nerve fibers are *cardioacceleratory:* stimulation through these fibers speeds the heartbeat by increasing the firing rate of the normal pacemaker (the S-A node) as well as of abnormal pacemakers (ectopic foci) in the various parts of the heart. Sympathetic stimulation also speeds the rate of conduction through the conducting system.

2. Parasympathetic fibers are *inhibitory:* stimulation of these fibers causes depression of pacemakers and slowing of conduction. Thus, with excessive parasympathetic (vagal) influence, the S-A node will slow its rate of discharge; conduction through the A-V node will also be slowed as a result of the vagal effect. (This latter phenomenon is exceedingly important in terms of A-V block and of digitalis effect—note it well and remember it. You will use it often.) Vagal stimulation also depresses ectopic pacemakers in the A-V node, a fact of great importance when nodal rhythms are being studied.

3. Vagal fibers do *not* reach the conducting tissues of the ventricles; vagal fibers reach and influence the S-A node, the atrial tissues generally, the A-V node, and probably the bundle of His, although this is not universally agreed. Sympathetic fibers, on the other hand, do reach all elements of the conducting system of the heart—atrial, A-V nodal, and ventricular.

Refractory period of conducting tissues (Fig. 1-3). Transmission of an electric wave, or potential, involves *work* on the part of cells doing the transmitting. Fatigue is produced, and the cells cannot transmit another impulse until they have recovered from this fatigue. The recovery of a particular tissue or cell takes a definite, measurable amount of time. The cell is said to have "recovered" when it is ready to transmit another impulse *normally.* It is said to have *partially recovered* when it is capable of transmission but is still somewhat fatigued so that the transmission is slow.

The time immediately following transmission of an impulse, during which a cell is not capable of any transmission at all, is called the absolute refractory period; in

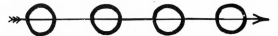

Transmitting activating impulse requires work on part of cells
involved

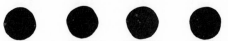

After passage of impulse, cells fatigued; not capable of another transmission at that instant

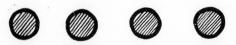

After short period of time, cells begin to recover—

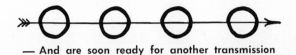

— And are soon ready for another transmission

Fig. 1-3. Refractory period—that is, period during which the cells of a conducting tissue are
unable to function because of fatigue from previous transmission.

other words, the cell is absolutely incapable of transmitting during this time. Following the absolute refractory period comes an interval of time when the cell is capable
of transmitting but does so *slowly*. This is the relative refractory period, when the rate
of transmission is slow relative to the normal rate.

Diseased cells almost always have an abnormally prolonged refractory period,
both relative and absolute. This is a fact of great clinical significance and will be referred to repeatedly throughout the text.

2 Basic facts and measurements in the electrocardiogram

NOMENCLATURE OF WAVES

The atrial deflection is called the P wave. An initial downward wave in the ventricular complex is a Q wave; any upward deflection is an R wave. Any downward deflection that follows an R wave is an S wave (Fig. 2-1, *A*).

TIME MEASUREMENTS

Each small square of the paper on which the electrocardiogram is recorded equals .04 second. Each large square contains five small ones and therefore equals .20 second.

Two measurements must be made at various times. The P-R interval, or the measurement from the first deflection of the P wave to the first deflection of the ventricular complex, is shown in Fig. 2-1, *B*. This is the time required for the activating wave to travel from the S-A node across the atria and through the A-V node and bundle of His. Normal values lie between .12 and .20 second.

Measurement of the QRS interval from the first ventricular deflection to the last (Fig. 2-1, *C*) demonstrates the time required for the spreading of the activating impulse through the ventricles from the bundle of His to the Purkinje fibers. Normal values are .09 second or less in the limb leads, .10 second or less in the precordial leads.

Some examples of normal electrocardiographic complexes are shown in Fig. 2-2.

Figs. 2-1 and 2-2 follow.

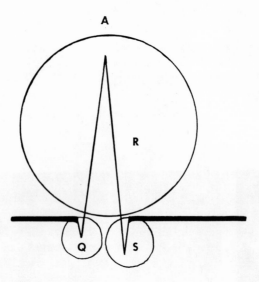

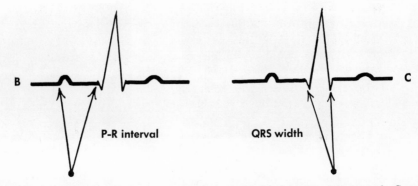

Fig. 2-1. A, Identity of ventricular deflections; **B,** method of measuring P-R interval; **C,** method of measuring the QRS interval.

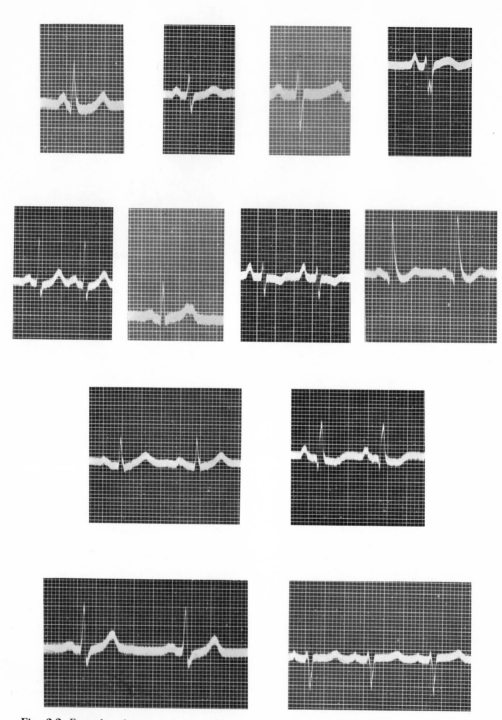

Fig. 2-2. Examples of normal electrocardiographic complexes. Practice measuring the time P-R and QRS intervals in each strip.

Part II
SIMPLE ARRHYTHMIAS

3 The sinus rhythms

"Sinus" refers to the sinoatrial node. Sinus rhythms are those rhythms that origi- nate in the S-A node—in other words, *normal* rhythms.

As a rule, a sinus rhythm produces a regular pulse that is obvious upon a bedside examination. This is not always the case, however. Some sinus rhythms may be quite irregular and on clinical examination may be confused with more serious arrhythmias.

Before going any further, the physician must be quite sure he can recognize a sinus rhythm in the electrocardiogram. *Read and reread this chapter.*

ELECTROCARDIOGRAPHIC DIAGNOSIS OF SINUS RHYTHMS

The S-A node discharges regularly. *P waves will therefore be inscribed at regular intervals.*

Each impulse travels down the A-V node and activates the ventricles. *Each P wave will therefore be followed at a regular interval by a ventricular complex.*

The reader will instantly ask: "How *long* is this regular interval?" To answer this question, it is necessary to remember only two numbers: .12 and .20. The time that elaspses from the origin of the beat (the beginning of the P wave) to the first deflec- tion of the ventricular complex will lie between these two figures. In other words, an impulse cannot follow a normal pathway from the S-A node to the ventricles and arrive there in less than .12 second. On the other hand, an impulse that takes longer than .20 second to traverse this pathway must have been slowed by diseased tissue along the way, probably in the A-V node. This interval is referred to as the P-R in- terval. (See Fig. 2-1, *B*, for the method of measurement.)

Each activating wave follows an identical pathway across the atria and through the ventricles. Therefore, the shape or contour of all complexes will be identical. Each P wave will look like every other P wave. Each ventricular complex will look exactly like every other ventricular complex (Fig. 3-1).

In summary, a normal or "sinus" mechanism is diagnosed when:

1. P waves appear at regular intervals.
2. Each P wave is followed at a regular normal interval by a ventricular complex.
3. All P waves and ventricular complexes have the same contour and configura- tion (Fig. 3-1).

VARIATIONS OF SINUS RHYTHMS

Sinus tachycardia (Fig. 3-2). In sinus tachycardia the rate is over 100. It will rarely exceed 160. Exertion, thyrotoxicosis, and fever are obvious causes.

Sinus bradycardia (Fig. 3-3). In sinus bradycardia the rate is under 60. It may drop to 40 or less in extreme cases.

Sinus arrhythmia (Fig. 3-4). In sinus arrhythmia the rhythm varies irregularly. Commonly, the rate becomes more rapid during inspiration and slows on expiration, although this is not always true. Sinus arrhythmias may fluctuate independently

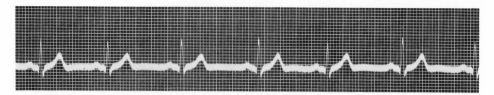

Fig. 3-1. Normal electrocardiogram.

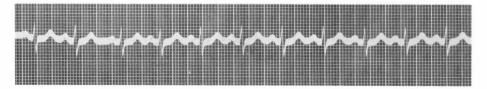

Fig. 3-2. Sinus tachycardia.

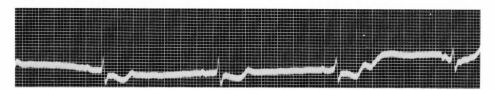

Fig. 3-3. Sinus bradycardia.

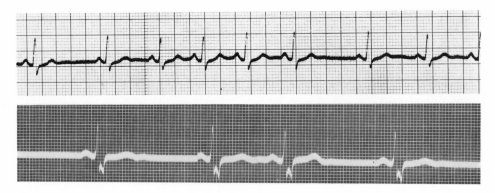

Fig. 3-4. Sinus arrhythmia.

of breathing. Even though the variation in rhythm is striking, it has no clinical significance.

Note that in each case the basic criteria for a sinus mechanism are present. Whether the beats come rapidly, slowly, or irregularly, each cycle consists of a P wave followed at a normal interval by a ventricular complex. The total configuration of each "beat" is exactly like that of every other "beat."

Complex disorders of S-A node function, such as the sick sinus syndrome and various forms of S-A block, are noted in Chapter 14.

4 Ectopic beats

The S-A node is the normal pacemaker of the heart, but it is not the only one. Hundreds of "extra" or "reserve" pacemakers are scattered through the subendocardium of the atria, the A-V node, and the ventricles. Any one of these bits of specialized myocardial tissue is capable of starting a beat. If the S-A node fails to fire or if its impulse fails to reach the ventricles, an ectopic pacemaker will discharge, thus performing its normal role of a "reserve," "standby," or "demand" pacemaker, ready to activate the heart if the normal mechanism fails. An ectopic beat thus produced is often called an "escape" beat; as the name implies, the ectopic pacemakers are normally suppressed or held in check by the activity of the S-A node. The passage of the normal activating wave across the heart discharges the ectopic pace-

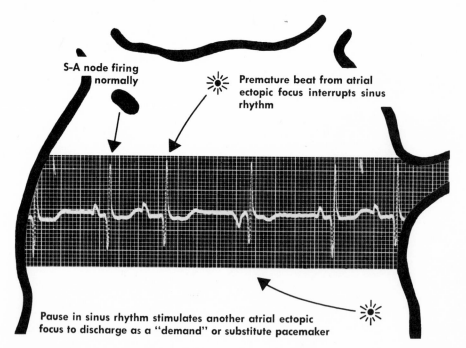

S-A node firing normally

Premature beat from atrial ectopic focus interrupts sinus rhythm

Pause in sinus rhythm stimulates another atrial ectopic focus to discharge as a "demand" or substitute pacemaker

Fig. 4-1. Types of firing of ectopic pacemakers. Notice the premature and "postmature" or escape firing of ectopic pacemaker in the atria. Premature firing is always abnormal and may be dangerous. Escape firing represents the physiologic function of an ectopic pacemaker.

makers before they have a chance to build up to the "firing level." When the normal activating mechanism fails, an ectopic pacemaker will escape—that is, it will fire because it is no longer suppressed. In other words, the ectopic pacemaker has "escaped" from the normal dominance of the S-A node and is free to discharge. When an ectopic pacemaker performs in this manner, it performs a physiologic and often a lifesaving function and should not be suppressed by the therapist.

Sometimes, on the other hand, an ectopic pacemaker becomes "irritable" and discharges even though the S-A node is functioning normally. This is the familiar "extrasystole," or premature ectopic beat. *Such premature beats are not physiologic and*

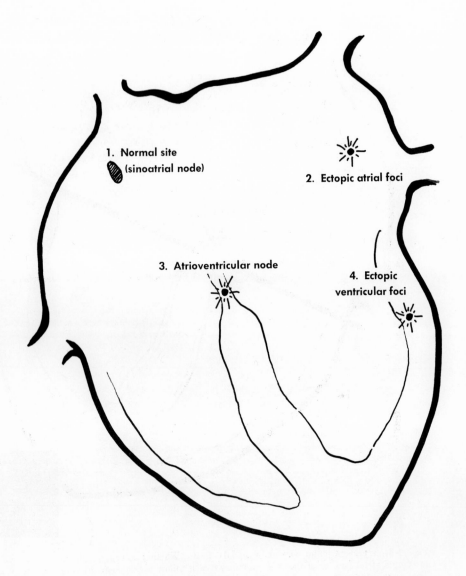

1. Normal site (sinoatrial node)

2. Ectopic atrial foci

3. Atrioventricular node

4. Ectopic ventricular foci

Fig. 4-2. A beat can originate in four different places. It is usually simple to recognize the origin of the beats. Clinically, it is important to differentiate between ventricular beats and those arising in the A-V node or atria. The way this is done is illustrated in Figs. 4-3 and 4-4.

serve no useful purpose: they may even threaten life. Fig. 4-1 illustrates these diametrically opposed activities arising in the ectopic pacemakers—on the one hand, escape beating, which is a physiologic and sometimes a lifesaving form of discharge, and, on the other, premature beating, an undesirable mechanism that can sometimes be dangerous. Throughout this text the words "escape ectopic beat" and "premature ectopic beat" will be used repeatedly. It is essential that the student have a thorough grasp of both concepts.

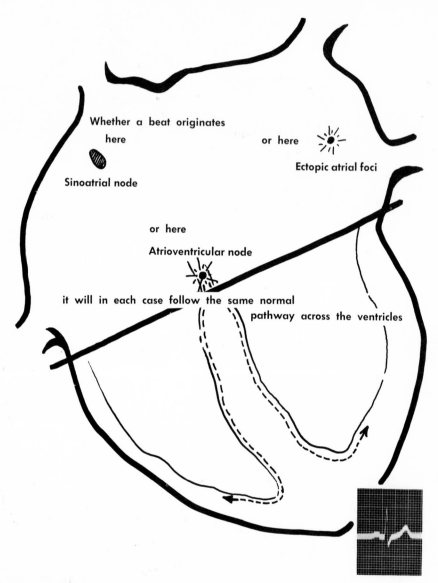

Fig. 4-3. Supraventricular (atrial or nodal) beats. Whether a beat originates at the S-A node, in ectopic atrial foci, or at the A-V junction, it will follow a normal pathway across the ventricles. The ventricular complex will therefore be normal. It is not vital to distinguish between atrial beats and nodal beats. The important thing is to distinguish between beats arising above the bifurcation of the bundle of His and those arising somewhere in the ventricles.

RECOGNIZING THE SITE OF ORIGIN OF AN ECTOPIC BEAT

The electrocardiogram will indicate the origin of an ectopic beat. By inspection of the tracing, one can tell whether an ectopic beat arises in the atria, the A-V node, or the ventricles. Figs. 4-2 to 4-5 illustrate the process by which this is done. *Identification of the site of origin of a beat is a skill that the physician must acquire for the diagnosis of all arrhythmias. Master this section of the book completely before going further.*

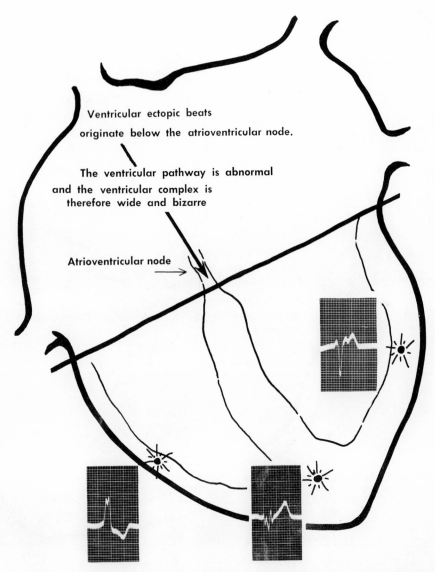

Fig. 4-4. Ventricular beats. If the beat originates anywhere below the point indicated by the arrow, the ventricular complex will be abnormal in contour. The impulse must travel a "backward" or eccentric path through the ventricles. The complex inscribed by such an impulse will therefore be wide and bizarre in shape. There will be no P wave preceding the ventricular complex. The shape of the ectopic ventricular beat is determined by the point of origin within the ventricles. Each ectopic focus has its own characteristic pattern.

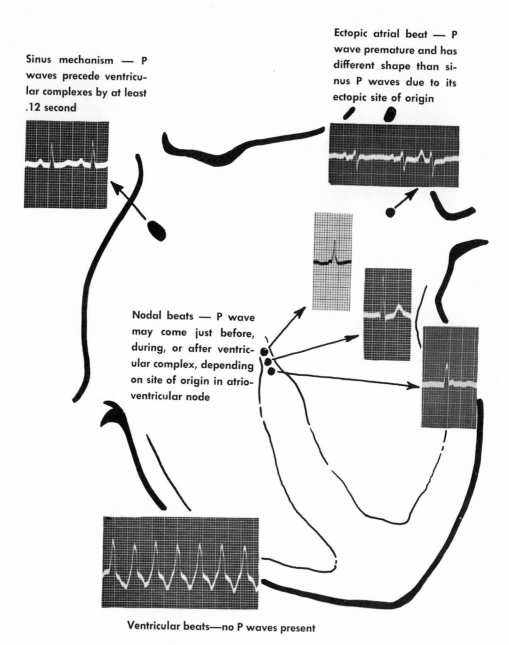

Sinus mechanism — P waves precede ventricular complexes by at least .12 second

Ectopic atrial beat — P wave premature and has different shape than sinus P waves due to its ectopic site of origin

Nodal beats — P wave may come just before, during, or after ventricular complex, depending on site of origin in atrioventricular node

Ventricular beats—no P waves present

Fig. 4-5. Relation of P waves to ventricular complex.

Atrial ectopic beats

Atrial premature beats

The electrocardiographic criteria for a diagnosis of premature atrial beats are simple and logical.

1. The beat appears prematurely.
2. The P wave of the premature beat has a different shape than the P wave of the sinus beat. This is a result of the abnormal pathway the exciting wave follows across the atria from the ectopic focus.
3. The P-R interval will lie in the normal range (.12 to .20 second).
4. The ventricular complex of the premature beat will be normal: the QRS-T, in other words, will be exactly like the QRS-T of the sinus beat, since the impulse from the ectopic focus comes down the normal pathway through the A-V node and across the ventricles.

In Fig. 4-6 the third and sixth beats are premature atrial beats. First, the beats are premature in time; second, the P waves of the premature beats differ in contour from the sinus P waves; and third, the ventricular complexes look exactly like those in the normal beats.

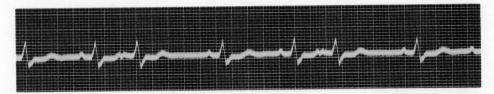

Fig. 4-6. Premature atrial beats.

Look closely at Fig. 4-7. The second and fifth beats are premature atrial beats. The premature P waves are partially buried in the preceding T wave, producing only a notch on the downstroke of the T. Sometimes premature P waves are completely buried in the preceding T wave and are not visible at all.

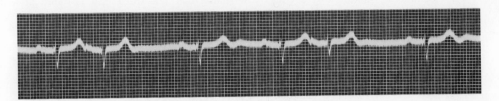

Fig. 4-7. Premature atrial beats.

Multiple premature atrial beats appearing in two's, three's, and whole "runs" may produce a grossly irregular pulse. Do not let the apparent complexity overwhelm you. Fig. 4-8 illustrates this kind of arrhythmia. Simply apply the same criteria and the diagnosis will be "sinus rhythm interrupted by frequent premature atrial beats." Note the premature atrial beats indicated by the arrows. In each beat the premature

P wave is completely buried in the preceding T: you can tell this by the difference in the shape of these T waves from the other T waves in the tracing.

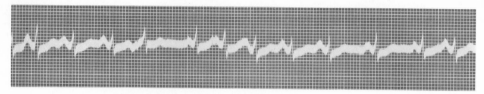

Fig. 4-8. Premature atrial beats.

In Fig. 4-9 atrial premature beats form a bigeminal rhythm. The second, fourth, and sixth beats are premature atrial complexes. The premature timing of the beats, the altered shape of the P wave, and the normal ventricular complexes are all well illustrated in this tracing. The inverted P waves are a common finding in ectopic atrial beats.

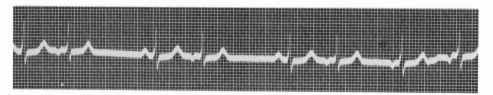

Fig. 4-9. Premature atrial beats.

Atrial escape ectopic beats

It is unusual for an ectopic focus in the atria to perform as an escape pacemaker, producing "postmature" beats. An example of this kind of firing is shown in Fig. 4-10. In the top strip *(A)*, the first beat has an upright P wave; following this beat there is a pause that is ended by a beat with an inverted P wave, followed at a normal conducting distance by a narrow, normal QRS. The third beat is identical with the second. In these two beats, an ectopic focus in the atrium has begun to discharge only because there was a delay or pause in the firing of the S-A node.

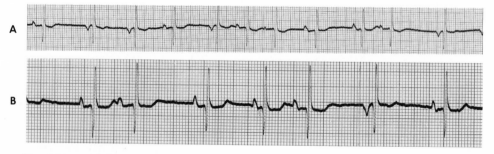

Fig. 4-10. A and **B,** Examples of premature and "postmature" firing from ectopic foci (see text).

Strip *B* shows both functions of an ectopic atrial pacemaker. The first beat is a normal sinus beat; the second is a typical premature atrial beat, followed by a pause. Two sinus beats follow, then a second premature atrial beat appears. The pause following this second premature beat ends with an atrial escape beat. Both premature and postmature firing of an atrial ectopic focus are illustrated in this strip. While this kind of escape or demand firing by an atrial pacemaker is relatively uncommon, the student must know that it can happen and must be prepared to recognize the phenomenon.

Atrioventricular nodal (junctional) beats

Recent investigation has shown that ectopic beats formerly thought to arise in the A-V node really arise in the junction of the A-V node with the atria or with the

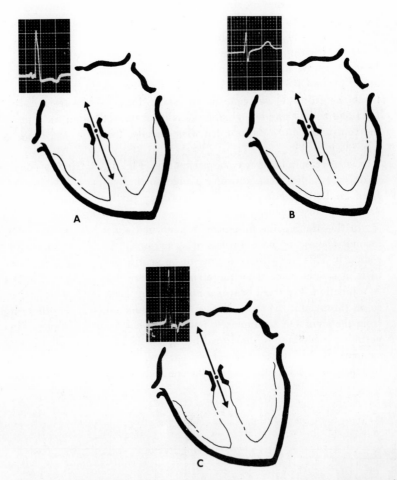

Fig. 4-11. Relation of P wave to QRS in A-V junctional beats. In **A,** transmission up into the atria takes place *before* transmission down into the ventricles from the A-V junctional focus. The atrial complex therefore comes just before the QRS. In **B,** the impulse from the A-V junction reaches the atria and the ventricles at the same time; as a result, the P wave is buried in the QRS and is usually not visible. In **C,** the A-V junctional impulse traveling down reaches the ventricles before the impulse traveling up reaches the atria. The P wave therefore follows the QRS.

bundle of His. It is probable that the cells of the A-V node proper do not have the capacity to generate beats; they only function as transmitters of impulses. The term "A-V junctional" has therefore come in to replace the older term "A-V nodal." From this point on in the text, the term "A-V junctional" will be used, since it is physiologically correct and will doubtless come to replace the older term in the near future.

When a beat arises in the A-V junction, it sends an impulse in two directions. One impulse moves from the junction *upward* across the atria. A second moves from the junctional focus down across the ventricles. The impulse moving down across the ventricles will follow the normal conducting pathway through the bundle of His and the bundle branches, so that the first characteristic of an A-V junctional beat will be a normal ventricular complex. *The word "normal" in this context means a QRS that is narrow (.10 second or less) and that looks like the complex of sinus beats.*

The second characteristic of an A-V junctional beat will be a retrograde atrial impulse—that is, one moving across the atria in a direction opposite to the normal exciting wave arising in the S-A node. This retrograde atrial impulse will appear just before, during, or after the QRS.

If the exciting wave moving upward from the junctional focus reaches the atria before the wave moving down reaches the ventricles, a P wave will be inscribed just ahead of the QRS (P-R interval will be less than .12 second). If the activating waves reach the atria and ventricles at the same time, the P wave will be "buried" in the QRS and will usually be invisible. Finally, if the activating wave penetrates *down* into the ventricles *before* the upward wave reaches the atria, the P wave will follow the QRS (Fig. 4-11).

Nodal ectopic beats may be premature (Fig. 4-12). Here a nodal ectopic beat appears every other beat, forming a bigeminal rhythm. (Bigeminy, of course, derives from the Latin *gemini*, twins. In describing rhythms, the term means a coupling or "twinning" of the pulse.)

In this tracing the first beat is a normal sinus beat with a P-R interval of .15 second. The second beat consists of a narrow QRS (.07 second) with no P wave preceding it. This beat is too narrow to be ventricular; since there is no P wave ahead of it, it cannot come from the atria; therefore, the only place it can arise is in the A-V junction. The third beat is a normal sinus beat, the fourth beat is junctional, and so on throughout the strip. Notice that the junctional beats differ slightly in contour from the sinus QRS complexes, with somewhat deeper S waves. This kind of minor variation is common in junctional beats, but the important point is that the ventricular complex of the junctional beats is narrow, indicating normal conduction from the junction down across the ventricular conducting system.

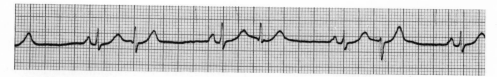

Fig. 4-12. A-V junctional ectopic focus forming a bigeminal rhythm. Note the normal sinus rhythm seen in every alternate beat of this strip. The beats appearing soon after each sinus beat are A-V junctional premature beats. They form a coupled or bigeminal rhythm. Note some degree of aberration, that is, different contour, in the QRS complexes of the junctional beats, particularly at the right-hand end of the strip.

Fig. 4-13 illustrates the escape or "postmature" firing of a junctional focus. In the first part of the strip there is a normal sinus rhythm interrupted by two junctional premature beats *(J)*. There is a long pause terminated by the beat marked *X*. In this beat the QRS complex is normal; no P wave precedes it; therefore, this beat must arise in the A-V junction. A retrograde P wave comes just after the QRS. Another junctional beat follows, with no visible P wave anywhere, and then, after another pause, two narrow QRS's are seen, again with no visible P waves. All these beats, of course, arise in the A-V junction and they illustrate both types of activity of a junctional ectopic pacemaker—premature or abnormal firing and postmature or physiologic functioning as a demand pacemaker.

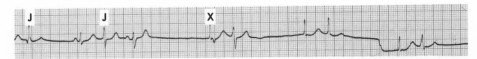

Fig. 4-13. Premature and "postmature" or escape firing of a junctional focus. Note the normal sinus beat at the left-hand side of this strip, followed by a premature A-V junctional beat. The pause following the second sinus beat is terminated by an A-V junctional beat. Note retrograde P wave following the QRS. The next six beats consist of an escape beat from the junctional focus, followed by a premature beat that also arises in the A-V junction. Thus an A-V junctional bigeminy is present for six beats.

Ventricular ectopic beats

Ventricular ectopic beats are easiest of all to recognize. They originate in the sub-endocardium of the ventricles below the bifurcation of the bundle of His. True ventricular ectopic beats move directly through myocardial tissue from the point of origin instead of down the specialized conducting tissue of the ventricles. The myocardium conducts slowly compared to the specialized conducting tissue. Speed of movement of an impulse through the myocardium varies from .5 to 1 meter per second, while the specialized conducting tissues conduct from 1 to 4 meters per second. The impulse moving directly through the myocardium from the ectopic focus in the ventricles, therefore, is like a car driving slowly over a bumpy dirt road, while transmission down the specialized conducting tissues can be compared to the same car driving along a freeway. The width of the ventricular complex of a ventricular ectopic beat reveals this slow movement: *any ectopic beat that arises in the ventricles will be .12 second wide in the adult heart. It will never be less.*

Since these ectopic beats follow a "backward" course across the ventricles, the QRS-T they produce will have a different shape from the QRS-T of a sinus impulse.

Finally, since ectopic beats arise in the ventricles, they are not initiated by a P wave.

Fig. 4-14 illustrates all these features of the ventricular ectopic beat. The second and next to last beats are typical ventricular ectopic beats with wide QRS, bizarre QRS-T, and absent P wave. Both these beats appear prematurely, interrupting a normal sinus rhythm; therefore, they represent the active pathologic discharge of a ventricular ectopic pacemaker.

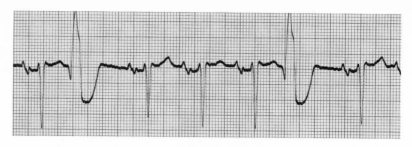

Fig. 4-14. Two ventricular ectopic beats from the same focus within the ventricles (see text).

Fig. 4-15 illustrates the phenomenon of ventricular bigeminy—that is, a basically normal sinus rhythm with a ventricular ectopic beat appearing every other beat. This figure also illustrates retrograde conduction from the ventricular ectopic focus up through the A-V node and into the atria. The retrograde P wave thus produced appears as a small notch on the ascending limb of the T wave of the ventricular ectopic beat. Recognition of a retrograde conduction from an ectopic focus up across the atria with production of a retrograde P wave is sometimes very important in analyzing arrhythmias.

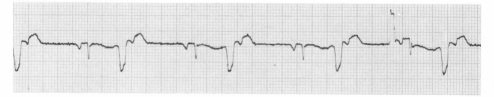

Fig. 4-15. Ventricular ectopic beats occurring every other beat, forming a bigeminal rhythm. Note retrograde P wave forming a notch in the upstroke of the T.

Ventricular beats arising in different foci have different contours. In fact, each ventricular ectopic focus has its own specific contour, as characteristic as a fingerprint. Under ordinary circumstances, a particular focus will always produce the same kind of ventricular complex. It is therefore easy to decide if more than one focus is firing in the ventricles: the QRS-T complexes of different ectopic foci will have different shapes. It is clinically important to recognize multifocal ventricular

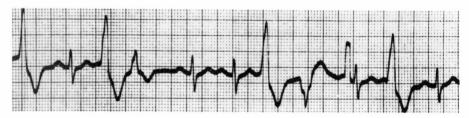

Fig. 4-16. Premature ventricular beats arising from multiple foci.

ectopic beats, since this is a common indication of widespread myocardial irritability. The first, third, seventh, and tenth beats shown in Fig. 4-16 are ventricular ectopic beats arising from a single focus. The fourth beat represents a different ectopic focus, and the eighth beat still another. Thus multifocal ventricular ectopic beats are present.

Escape ventricular ectopic beats

Fig. 4-17 is an example of a ventricular ectopic focus firing in its normal role as an escape or demand pacemaker. Just as in the junctional and atrial escape beats previously illustrated, the ventricular escape here is performing a useful function: had it not fired, there would have been no systole for what might have been a dangerously long time.

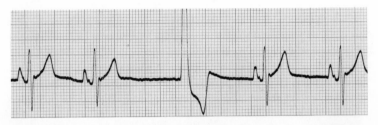

Fig. 4-17. An escape or "postmature" beat arising from a ventricular focus.

CLINICAL ASPECTS
Bedside diagnosis

Premature ectopic beats are usually apparent on counting the pulse or listening to the heartbeat. When they occur rapidly or irregularly or in large numbers, the rhythm may become so confusing that an electrocardiogram will be the only source of exact diagnosis. It is sometimes stated that on auscultation, supraventricular ectopic beats (atrial and A-V junctional) have a more nearly normal sound than ventricular ectopic beats, but this phenomenon is not sufficiently reliable to permit accurate differentiation of the two types of beat. Inspection of the jugular venous pulsations may, in very expert hands, sometimes provide a clue to the site of origin of an ectopic beat. Again, even in the best hands, this is not a precise mode of diagnosis, and, for most physicians, it is not practical at all.

Compensatory pause

Usually, although not always, there will be a pause following a premature beat. This pause has given rise to a great deal of confusion quite needlessly, since the postectopic pause—often loosely referred to as the "compensatory pause"—is, first, a very simple phenomenon and, second, of very little practical use.

There is a pause following almost all atrial ectopic beats because the ectopic impulse, as it traverses the atria, discharges the tissue in the S-A node that had been building up for the next normal sinus beat. As a result, the S-A node has to "start over" building up a charge for another beat; there is therefore a delay before the next discharge. Compare the S-A node to a workman who stacks up blocks of concrete that are loaded into a conveyor. Imagine that the workman has to stack ten blocks before the unit is ready to be loaded on the conveyor. Now imagine that somebody comes along and knocks over his stack of blocks when it is only six blocks high. The workman will have to start over with block one to assemble a new unit, and, naturally, his delivery time for the next unit will be late. This is like the mechanism by which an ectopic atrial impulse produces a delay in the appearance of the next sinus beat.

When a junctional ectopic beat is conducted retrogradely across the atria, the same thing happens, and there is a pause for the same reason.

The ventricular ectopic beat can produce a pause in one of two ways. First, the sinus P wave fires on time but it does so while the ventricular ectopic beat is spreading across the ventricles. As a result, the P wave is "buried" in the QRS and is not visible. Further, when the atrial impulse reaches the A-V node, it encounters tissues that have already been discharged by the ventricular ectopic beat and cannot conduct the S-A impulse. There is therefore a pause until the next sinus beat crosses the atria and is conducted through the A-V node to the ventricles. This will be a "full" compensatory pause, meaning that the sinus beat following the ventricular premature beat appears when it would have if there had been no ventricular premature beat and if there had been, instead, a normally conducted sinus beat. In other words, the interval from the P wave before the ventricular ectopic beat to the one after it will be double the normal P-P interval. This is called a "full" compensatory pause.

If the ventricular ectopic beat is conducted retrogradely through the A-V node and across the atria, it will discharge the S-A node and produce a pause in exactly the same way that atrial and junctional beats do.

Thus, a compensatory pause may be "full" or less than "full" following a ventricular ectopic beat and will almost always be less than "full" (two normal P-P intervals) following junctional or atrial beats. For this reason, the duration of the compensatory pause is not much use in localizing ectopic beats.

5 Sustained ectopic rhythms

Instead of firing a single beat, an ectopic focus may continue to discharge, setting the rhythm of the heart for minutes, hours, or days. There are two kinds of continuous or sustained ectopic rhythms, just as there are two kinds of single ectopic beats.

Active ectopic rhythms. Instead of a single premature beat, the "irritable" ectopic focus may continue firing, producing a rapid, regular run of premature beats. This is paroxysmal tachycardia. Like premature beats, paroxysmal tachycardia is always abnormal and is sometimes dangerous.

"Escape" or "passive" ectopic rhythms. Like single escape beats, these rhythms appear when the S-A node fails to perform adequately. Because of lack of stimulation from the normal pacemaker, the ectopic pacemaker will continue firing in the slow-to-normal range, functioning as a demand pacemaker and often saving the patient's life. These relatively slow, regular ectopic rhythms are called "idioventricular" or "idionodal," depending on the location of the ectopic pacemaker. (It is rare for an atrial escape rhythm to appear, but when it does, "idioatrial" would be the proper and consistent term.) Escape or "idio" rhythms represent the physiologic function of an ectopic focus; suppressive drugs should never be used to eradicate such a rhythm. Therapy should be directed toward restoring normal S-A function if possible.

PAROXYSMAL TACHYCARDIA

Characteristically, paroxysmal tachycardia starts and stops abruptly. *During the tachycardia, the rate is constant;* breathing, change in position, anxiety, or any of the other factors that would change the rate of a sinus tachycardia will have no effect on paroxysmal tachycardia.

If a physician sees a patient whose heart is beating rapidly with a regular rhythm, if the rate is between approximately 160 and 280, and if the onset of the rapid, regular rhythm has been abrupt, the physician is likely to be dealing with a paroxysmal tachycardia. *The physician must still take an electrocardiogram before attempting therapy, for several reasons:*

It must be established that paroxysmal tachycardia is actually present, instead of, for example, flutter or atrial tachycardia with A-V block. The electrocardiogram is the only way to make this kind of differentiation.

It is essential to determine the origin of the paroxysmal tachycardia—atrial, junctional, or ventricular—for both prognostic and therapeutic reasons. There is absolutely no way of differentiating atrial, junctional, and ventricular paroxysmal tachycardia with acceptable accuracy on clinical grounds.

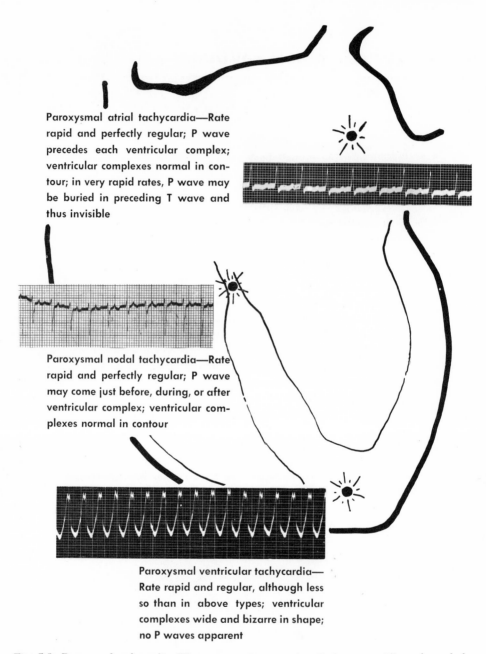

Paroxysmal atrial tachycardia—Rate rapid and perfectly regular; P wave precedes each ventricular complex; ventricular complexes normal in contour; in very rapid rates, P wave may be buried in preceding T wave and thus invisible

Paroxysmal nodal tachycardia—Rate rapid and perfectly regular; P wave may come just before, during, or after ventricular complex; ventricular complexes normal in contour

Paroxysmal ventricular tachycardia— Rate rapid and regular, although less so than in above types; ventricular complexes wide and bizarre in shape; no P waves apparent

Fig. 5-1. Paroxysmal tachycardia. When an ectopic pacemaker discharges rapidly and regularly, paroxysmal tachycardia is the result. Like premature beats, the tachycardias can originate in the atria, A-V junction, or the ventricles. The three types are differentiated by applying the same criteria one applies to premature beats. The rate may vary from 140 to 300 or more beats per minute in any type of paroxysmal tachycardia.

Atrial and atrioventricular junctional tachycardia
Electrocardiogram recognition

Atrial and A-V junctional tachycardia are often lumped together as "supraventricular" paroxysmal tachycardia. This is a sensible classification, since it is often impossible to tell them apart and since the two rhythms are very similar in many ways in terms of prognosis and treatment. Electrocardiographic diagnosis is based on the simplest kind of reasoning.

A narrow QRS (.09 second in the limb leads, .10 second in the precordial leads) can be produced *only* by a supraventricular impulse—that is, one arising in the atrial and A-V junction and following a normal rapid course down through the ventricular conducting tissues. Therefore, if the ECG records a perfectly regular rate (160 to 280) with narrow QRS complexes, the presumptive diagnosis is *supraventricular paroxysmal tachycardia.*

If P waves are present at a normal conducting distance before each QRS complex (P-R .12 to .20 second), the diagnosis is *paroxysmal atrial tachycardia.*

If no P waves are visible, the rhythm may be either atrial or nodal. At such rapid rates as these, the P wave is often hidden in the preceding T wave. Therefore, the diagnosis, when the tracing records rapid, regular, narrow QRS complexes without P waves, is simply supraventricular tachycardia. (This may be either atrial or A-V junctional.)

If abnormally shaped (retrograde) P waves appear just before or just after the QRS complexes, the diagnosis is A-V junctional tachycardia.

In other words, use exactly the same criteria you would for a single ectopic beat.

The last four ventricular complexes shown in Fig. 5-2 are normal sinus beats. Now inspect the other complexes in the tracing. Note that they are rapid and regular. The ventricular complexes are narrow and look exactly like the ventricular complexes of the sinus beats; therefore, these rapid, regular beats are either atrial or nodal—that is, they are supraventricular. A P wave precedes each ventricular complex, with a P-R interval of .16 second; therefore, the beats come from an ectopic atrial focus. The strip shows the end of a paroxysm of atrial tachycardia, with a resumption of normal sinus rhythm.

Fig. 5-3 shows typical paroxysmal atrial tachycardia. The rate is 170. The ventricular complexes are normal (narrow) and the P waves appear about .12 second before each ventricular complex. In other words, the criteria for an atrial beat are fulfilled in each complex.

Inspect Fig. 5-4. Note the normal appearance of the ventricular complexes. No P waves are present, or at least none are visible. This paroxysm of tachycardia *probably* arises in the A-V nodal junction, since the criteria for a junctional beat are fulfilled—*normal, narrow, ventricular complexes and no P waves.* Note the use of the word "probably." One cannot be sure there are not P waves buried in each preceding T wave. This is not crucial, clinically, since atrial and A-V junctional tachycardia are in many respects identical in prognosis and treatment.

Sinus tachycardia may resemble paroxysmal atrial tachycardia in the electrocardiogram. There are some clinical features of the two arrhythmias that will help in this differentiation (see p. 34). The *shape* of the atrial complexes seen during paroxysmal atrial tachycardia will be clearly different from the shape of the normal sinus P waves, if the physician is fortunate enough to have a previous tracing with which to compare it.

In Fig. 5-5 a different P wave relationship appears. Note the short, spiked P wave *following* each ventricular complex. This means that the beat arises in the A-V nodal junction. (Criteria for diagnosis of an A-V junctional beat here are presence of normal, narrow, ventricular complexes, with P wave following a QRS. This is therefore paroxysmal A-V junctional tachycardia.)

For clinical purposes, it is well to remember that atrial and A-V junctional tachycardia are usually identical in prognosis and treatment. Often they cannot be differentiated by any means. The diagnosis of *paroxysmal supraventricular tachy-*

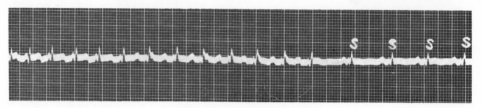

Fig. 5-2. Paroxysmal tachycardia.

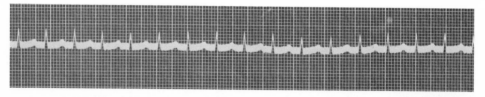

Fig. 5-3. Paroxysmal atrial tachycardia.

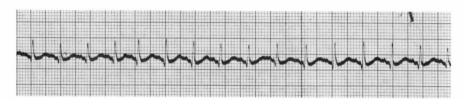

Fig. 5-4. Paroxysmal supraventricular tachycardia. This may be atrial or nodal in origin. P waves may be "hidden" in the preceding T waves.

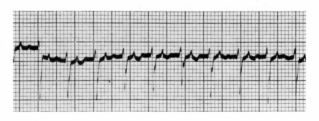

Fig. 5-5. Paroxysmal nodal tachycardia. P waves follow the QRS complexes.

cardia is frequently sufficient for all practical purposes. Paroxysmal supraventricular tachycardia does not necessarily connote organic heart disease and it often occurs in individuals without other evidence of cardiac pathology.

Ventricular tachycardia

Ventricular tachycardia is much more serious than the other types. It almost always connotes organic heart disease, usually severe. Proper diagnosis in these cases may well be of life or death significance.

Ventricular tachycardia is recognized in the same manner as ventricular ectopic beats. Inspect Fig. 5-6. Note that the rate is rapid (150) and regular. The ventricular complexes are wide (.16 second) and bizarre in shape. No P waves are present. The presumptive diagnosis, therefore, is paroxysmal ventricular tachycardia.

Fig. 5-7 illustrates a common finding in patients with ventricular tachycardia. Notice the spiked, small complexes marked *Pr* in this strip. These are *retrograde P waves*—that is, they are produced by the impulse arising in the ventricles and traveling *backward* up the A-V node and into the atria. (Notice that in this tracing this happens every other beat, for a time, with some regularity.) Retrograde P waves are fairly common in ventricular tachycardia. Often these retrograde P waves will

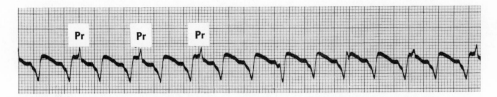

Fig. 5-6. Ventricular tachycardia.

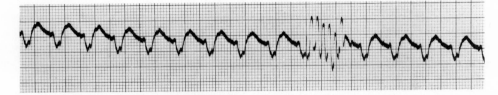

Fig. 5-7. Ventricular tachycardia with intermittent retrograde conduction to atria (*Pr*).

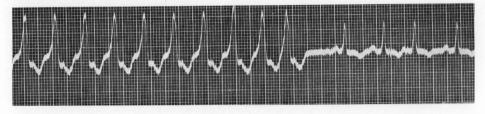

Fig. 5-8. End of ventricular tachycardia and resumption of normal sinus rhythm.

appear as small humps or spikes in the T wave. Some degree of *block* to these retrograde beats is common, since "backward" conduction through the A-V node seems to be relatively difficult. The abnormal P waves may appear with every beat, every other beat, every third beat, or at completely irregular intervals.

The end of a paroxysm of ventricular tachycardia and the resumption of normal sinus rhythm is illustrated in Fig. 5-8. The difference between the configuration of the ectopic ventricular complexes and the sinus beats is obvious. Notice that the last two ventricular complexes of the paroxysmal tachycardia are closer together than all the others. This is fairly common and the reason for it is not completely understood.

Clinical manifestations

The onset of a paroxysmal tachycardia will almost always be accompanied by symptoms of "pounding of the heart," acute apprehension, and sometimes breathlessness. Remember that a bout of paroxysmal tachycardia is a frightening experience, particularly the first time.

The pulse, as well as the apical beat, will be rapid and regular. This is common to many arrhythmias and is not diagnostic.

Vagal stimulation

Vagal stimulation by proper massage of the carotid sinus will sometimes end a supraventricular paroxysmal tachycardia. It will *not* affect a ventricular tachycardia. (Remember, the vagal fibers do not reach the conducting tissues of the ventricles.)

If vagal stimulation works at all in paroxysmal tachycardia, it works abruptly— the arrhythmia ends at once. There are no exceptions to this rule. To put it another way, vagal stimulation will *never* produce transient slowing of the rate when paroxysmal tachycardia is present. The rhythm either stops completely and abruptly or it is not affected at all. This "all-or-none" phenomenon contrasts with the effect of vagal stimulation in sinus tachycardia, when the rate often slows transiently and then speeds again.

Clinical differentiation of sinus tachycardia from paroxysmal tachycardia

Sinus tachycardia and paroxysmal supraventricular tachycardia may look identical on the electrocardiogram. They can be differentiated by some simple clinical observations:

1. The difference in vagal effect, as noted previously, may be diagnostic.
2. Onset of sinus tachycardia is almost never abrupt: the rate gradually builds up, whereas paroxysmal tachycardia starts abruptly.
3. External influence, such as exercise, posture, breathing, relaxing, and the like, will affect the rate in sinus tachycardia, whereas these maneuvers will have no effect on the rate in paroxysmal tachycardia.

Therapy

Treatment varies with the *kind* of tachycardia present. An electrocardiogram should always be recorded first, for the reasons outlined earlier in this chapter. If for some reason an electrocardiogram cannot be recorded, vagal stimulation should be tried. This can do no harm and may end the episode promptly. Many patients learn to use various forms of vagal stimulation, such as retching, straining, swallowing ice water rapidly, and so on. These maneuvers are often effective.

If vagal stimulation fails, do not administer further treatment until an electrocardiogram can be recorded. If an electrocardiogram is completely out of reach, the tachycardia should be treated as though it were a ventricular tachycardia. The rationale here is that the treatment for ventricular tachycardia will do no harm in supraventricular tachycardia—some types of treatment directed at ventricular tachycardia will end supraventricular tachycardia. On the other hand, digitalis, the chief mode of treatment in supraventricular tachycardia, is very dangerous in ventricular tachycardia.

Supraventricular tachycardia

SYMPATHOMIMETIC DRUGS. *Phenylephrine hydrochloride (Neo-Synephrine)*, 0.5 mg. intravenously, is a useful drug and often terminates supraventricular tachycardia. The dose may be repeated or even doubled *if blood pressure does not rise dangerously.*

The effectiveness of sympathomimetic drugs in terminating supraventricular tachycardia is associated with the rise in blood pressure that accompanies their administration. A controlled rise in systolic pressure, to the range of 160 to 170, is therefore the goal of treatment. This can also be accomplished by giving the drug in an intravenous drip with 5 mg of Neo-Synephrine in 100 to 250 ml of 5% glucose in water.

WARNING: Sympathomimetic drugs may be dangerous. Patients with coronary artery disease, hypertension, or any degree of A-V block should not be given sympathomimetic drugs. The patient who exhibits a very slow sinus rate are when not in paroxysmal tachycardia should not be given sympathomimetic drugs, since dangerous slowing may take place.

The ideal candidate, for example, would be a 20-year-old female in vigorous health without history of heart disease who had a first attack of paroxysmal supraventricular tachycardia. In a 45-year-old male suffering his first attack, the drug should not be used, since the chances, statistically, that such a person would have some degree of coronary artery disease are excellent.

Vagomimetic drugs. Neostigmine (Prostigmin), 1 mg, may be given subcutaneously for vagal effect. Carotid sinus stimulation after injection (10 to 20 minutes) may produce a "summated" vagus effect that may terminate the arrhythmias. Remember the usual contraindications and warnings about Prostigmin—don't give it to patients with bronchial asthma, and always have atropine on hand for the occasional patient who will overreact with a cholinergic crisis. If a nurse is watching the patient, be sure to instruct her carefully about the clinical manifestations of a vagal overreaction and be sure atropine has been ordered to be given, if needed.

Edrophonium (Tensilon) is another vagomimetic drug that has shown promise in the treatment of supraventricular tachycardias. More clinical evaluation is needed; at this point, it can be stated only that the drug seems promising.

Digitalis. Digitalis glycosides are considered by many to be the best source of treatment. *Digoxin (Lanoxin)* is given in divided doses, orally or intramuscularly. The total amount required will vary a great deal—older patients will take much less digitalis than younger ones, on an average, and it is best to divide the doses into 0.25-mg increments, giving them every 3 or 4 hours until a total of 1 to 1.5 mg has been administered.

Note that intravenous administration has not been mentioned. In my opinion intravenous digitalis is used much more often that it should be; supraventricular tachycardia rarely threatens life. In a severely ill cardiac patient, such a tachycardia may indeed be dangerous and extreme measures are justified to terminate it, but in most cases the arrhythmia will be tolerated well for hours or days, and the physician is not justified in resorting to dangerous means of therapy to end it.

If intravenous digoxin is to be given, it should be given very slowly; 0.25 mg should be injected over a 15-minute interval. Injections should not be faster, since a dangerous concentration of the drug accumulates in the heart very abruptly.

Deslanoside, 1.6 mg, may be given intravenously in divided doses. The same caution about *slow* administration applies; so does the same precaution about intravenous administration of any digitalis preparation.

Quinidine and procainamide. In resistant cases, either of these drugs may be used in the manner and doses outlined for ventricular tachycardia. Quinidine in particular is very effective in supraventricular paroxysmal tachycardia.

Diphenylhydantoin (Dilantin). Diphenylhydantoin, in my experience, is of little use in these arrhythmias.

Propranolol (Inderal). Propranolol or any of the other beta adrenergic blocking agents are sometimes effective but should never be used without consultation by a trained cardiologist. Intractable and often lethal failure may be precipitated by use of these drugs; they should be administered only by those very skilled in their use. (See Chapter 19.)

Electroshock. Synchronized cardioversion is very effective in terminating supraventricular paroxysmal tachycardias. Again, if possible, a physician skilled and experienced in this form of treatment should be called in consultation for the electroversion, since the method does present hazards and one who is not thoroughly familiar with the complications and contraindications may do more harm than good. Very bizarre arrhythmias often appear immediately after electroversion, and, of course, use of electroversion in a patient who has been taking digitalis is particularly hazardous.

Ventricular tachycardia

First, a warning! *Do not use digitalis preparations of any kind in treating patients with ventricular tachycardia!* The ventricular rate often increases rapidly, and the ventricles may fibrillate after exhibition of digitalis or digitalis-like compounds.

A few authors have minimized this danger on the basis of a small number of cases in which disaster did not strike. I have seen patients with ventricular tachycardia whose lives were endangered because of the administration of digitalis compounds, in one case increasing the pulse to a rate too rapid to count.

Lidocaine (Xylocaine). Lidocaine may be given by direct intravenous push with a bolus of about 75 mg at a time, or it may be given by drip. I prefer to administer 75 to 100 mg of lidocaine by intravenous push, repeating the procedure three or four times at about 6-minute intervals. If there is no response, intravenous drip with 1 gm of lidocaine in 500 ml of 5% dextrose in water may be tried, regulating the drip so that the patient receives about 2 or 3 mg of the drug per minute (range:

1 to 4 mg per minute). If the arrhythmia has not responded in 2 hours or if the patient's condition deteriorates, procainamide should then be used.

Procainamide (Pronestyl). Procainamide is administered intravenously for the most rapid effect. The dose required to halt the tachycardia may be as little as 200 mg or as much as 2,000 mg. Since the chief toxic effect of procainamide is an abrupt lowering of the blood pressure, it is wise to administer the drug by drip with a Y-tube connection to a reservoir of a pressor amine that can be introduced if needed.

I usually begin treatment with 1 gm of procainamide dissolved in 500 ml of 5% glucose in water. The rate of drip may be rapid initially (120 drops per minute) and may be slowed when conversion is achieved or when blood pressure begins to fall. Blood pressure must be checked frequently during intravenous administration, and the pressor agent should be added to the drip as soon as a significant fall is detected. This dose may be repeated two or three times in a 24-hour period if necessary.

If the ventricular tachycardia does not appear to threaten life, oral procainamide may be employed. A large initial dose of 1 to 1.25 gm is used, followed in 2 hours by 0.5 gm. Doses of 0.5 to 0.75 gm may be given every 2 hours until conversion is achieved. Although the oral route is relatively slow, it is safer in terms of maintenance of normal blood pressure.

Intramuscular administration of 0.25 gm of procainamide at 2- or 4-hour intervals may also terminate the arrhythmia. To maintain a normal rhythm once achieved, oral or intramuscular doses of approximately 0.25 gm four times a day may be employed.

Quinidine. Since the introduction of procainamide, lidocaine, and synchronized electrocardioversion, quinidine has fallen into disuse in ventricular tachycardia. However, oral quinidine, suitably employed, can be remarkably effective, and the physician should at least be familiar with dosage schedules in ventricular tachycardia.

If other medications have failed and if electroversion is not available, quinidine may well be worth trying. (I have converted many cases of ventricular tachycardia to sinus rhythm with quinidine in years past.)

I begin treatment with an oral dose of 0.2 gm hourly and I may continue this dose for 8 to 12 hours. There is good laboratory and clinical evidence to suggest that hourly dosage of quinidine maintains a better blood and tissue level of the drug than the 2- or 4-hour intervals formerly used. After 3 hours, the physician should check carefully for evidence of toxicity. If there is no nausea or vomiting, if the blood pressure is not unduly depressed, and if the ventricular tachycardia persists, a total dose of 2 to 4 gm of quinidine may be administered, in divided doses, in a 24-hour period. These doses may be given every hour, every 2 hours, or every 4 hours, as the physician deems advisable.

Quinidine should never be administered intravenously. Before modern modes of therapy became available, there were rare indications for such use; now it is never justified. Intravenous quinidine is very dangerous and many deaths have followed its use.

Intramuscular quinidine is about as safe as oral quinidine; doses of 100 mg given at about the same intervals as outlined for oral dosage may be very effective.

After a sinus mechanism has been restored, 0.2 gm of quinidine given three times a day may be effective in maintaining a normal rhythm.

Chronic toxic effects of quinidine include nausea, vomiting, A-V block, intra-ventricular block, and ventricular standstill. Patients taking quinidine must be checked frequently for evidence of toxicity.

When time permits, it is wise to administer a relatively small dose of quinidine (0.1 gm) initially, since some patients will manifest an idiosyncrasy to quinidine that will become obvious within 2 hours of administration of this test dose.

Electroversion. Electroversion, again, is a very effective mode of therapy in ventricular tachycardia. Warnings are again sounded: the electroversion should be under the supervision of a skilled physician who has had wide experience in treat-ment of cardiac arrhythmias. Electroversion should not be used when the patient has been taking digitalis or when there is a question of a digitalis-toxic arrhythmia (see Chapter 10). The general practitioner or the internist without special cardiologic training would do well to seek consultation before using cardioversion in these cases, since some very bizarre and dangerous complications may ensue.

"ESCAPE" OR "PASSIVE" ECTOPIC RHYTHMS

Under certain conditions, the S-A node will become depressed and stop discharg-ing, or it may discharge so slowly that the cardiac rate becomes inadequate. Life is then maintained by the ectopic pacemakers of the heart, usually those in the A-V junction or in the ventricles (Fig. 5-9).

Acute hypoxia, severe myocardial damage, and reflex activity through the vagus nerve are the common causes of depression of the S-A node. Clinically, these may be seen in patients with shock, acute carditis, anesthesia, or myocardial infarction.

Whatever the cause, the escape or junctional rhythm appears as a lifesaving mechanism, in contrast to the dangerous abnormal discharge of a paroxysmal tachy-cardia. Electrocardiographic criteria for diagnosis of escape ectopic rhythms are exactly the same as in isolated ectopic beats or paroxysmal tachycardias.

Clinical diagnosis is particularly difficult in these rhythms, since they are quite regular and are frequently in the normal range. Unless the physician is an extraor-dinarily skilled cardiologist, he will not be able to detect these rhythms or even suspect their presence unless an electrocardiogram is being recorded.

Fig. 5-10 is a good example of an intermittent escape ectopic rhythm that appears when the S-A node fails to discharge. In the top strip, there is a run of normal sinus rhythm in the beats marked *S*. After the fourth sinus beat there is a pause; three beats are then noted, which appear at a slower rate. These beats present a narrow QRS complex and hence are supraventricular; since there are no P waves, the beats must arise in the A-V nodal junction. The rate is 68, in contrast to the sinus rate, which is approximately 100 beats per minute. Note in the two strips how the slower A-V junctional escape rhythm "picks up" whenever the sinus node fails to discharge. In Fig. 5-11 a junctional rhythm is present throughout. The rate is approximately 68, the rhythm is regular, the QRS complexes are narrow, and no P waves are noted. Here the patient's life literally depends on the presence of an ectopic pace-maker in the A-V nodal junction, since there is no evidence of atrial activity at all—that is, no P waves are present.

The range of these escape rhythms is wide, from as little as 38 or 40 beats per minute to slightly over 100. This range has led to some confusion in terminology. It is common to use the words "idioventricular" or "idionodal" for the slower rates and to use "idioventricular tachycardia" or "idionodal tachycardia" for rates in the normal range—at 100 or slightly over. "Accelerated idio rhythms" also describes the latter category. This is perfectly acceptable as long as the physician does not confuse these slow, regular rhythms with paroxysmal tachycardia.

Fig. 5-12 illustrates a typical idioventricular rhythm. The rate is slow (75), the QRS complexes are wide, and there are no P waves preceding the ventricular complexes. Note the notching in the T wave of each beat in this tracing. This notch,

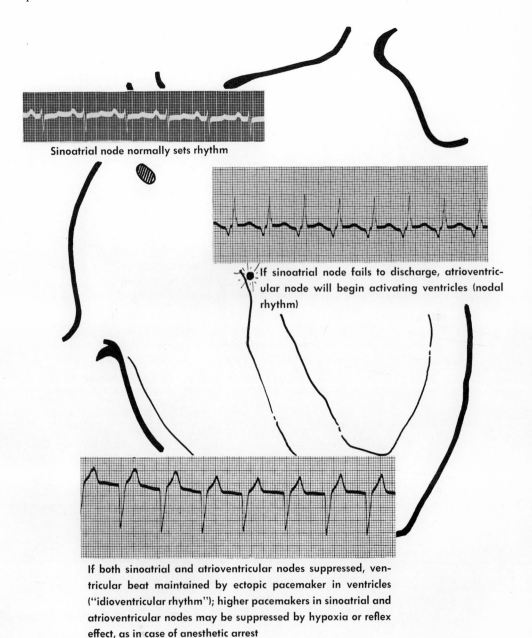

Sinoatrial node normally sets rhythm

If sinoatrial node fails to discharge, atrioventricular node will begin activating ventricles (nodal rhythm)

If both sinoatrial and atrioventricular nodes suppressed, ventricular beat maintained by ectopic pacemaker in ventricles ("idioventricular rhythm"); higher pacemakers in sinoatrial and atrioventricular nodes may be suppressed by hypoxia or reflex effect, as in case of anesthetic arrest

Fig. 5-9. Sustained escape rhythms arising in the A-V junction and in the ventricles ("idionodal" and "idioventricular" rhythms).

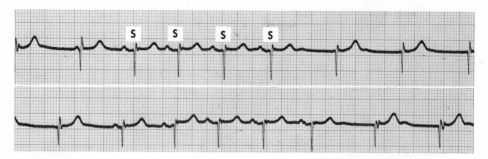

Fig. 5-10. Escape ectopic rhythm arising in A-V junction. Note intermittent appearance of a slow regular rhythm with narrow QRS complexes *not* preceded by P waves. The A-V junction "escapes" intermittently because of a pause in the discharge of the S-A node.

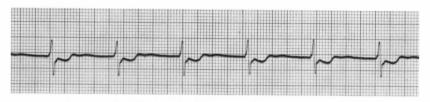

Fig. 5-11. A-V junctional rhythm. Note characteristic narrow QRS complexes not preceded by P waves appearing in a slow, regular rhythm.

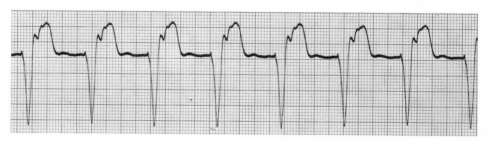

Fig. 5-12. Idioventricular rhythm. Note retrograde conduction to atria with inverted P wave on ascending limb of T waves.

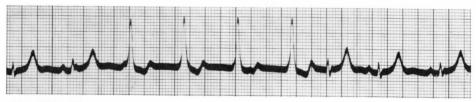

Fig. 5-13. Idioventricular rhythm interrupting normal sinus rhythm. Idioventricular rate of 82 puts this in the class of "accelerated" idioventricular rhythm.

in each case, represents a retrograde P wave; the ventricular complex has moved upward through the A-V node and across the atria, discharging the S-A node. This idioventricular rhythm is probably present because of the retrograde conduction across the atria. In other words, the retrograde P waves are coming up the A-V node and across the atria from the ventricular ectopic focus just fast enough to keep the S-A node discharged.

Fig. 5-13 shows a four-beat run of an idioventricular rhythm interrupting a normal sinus rhythm. The first three beats on the tracing are normal sinus beats. The next four are wide, slow beats not preceded by P waves. The rate of the idioventricular rhythm is 68, while the sinus rate is 88.

This figure gives the reader a chance to reason. Notice that the P-R interval of the first normal sinus beat following the end of the idioventricular rhythm is longer than the others. Why? The assumption is that the ventricular ectopic beats have been penetrating the A-V node for some distance, even though they are not reaching the atria. This *concealed conduction* up the A-V node fatigues the A-V nodal tissue so that the first P-R interval coming close on the heels of this kind of concealed conduction will be abnormally prolonged.

Treatment

Treatment of escape ectopic rhythms depends entirely on the cause of the "escape."

Inadequate rate of discharge of S-A node (sinus bradycardia, S-A block, sinus pauses). When the S-A node is discharging so slowly that an ectopic focus escapes and sets up a sustained slow ectopic rhythm, therapy is directed at speeding the S-A node, if possible. Medical therapy is based on atropine and isoproterenol. From .5 to 1 mg of atropine, given intravenously or subcutaneously, will often speed the S-A node to adequate rates, thereby suppressing the ectopic pacemaker. The atropine may be repeated as often as the side effects of the drug permit or as the physician thinks wise. (Remember: glaucoma and urinary retention are both contraindications to the use of atropine.)

Isoproterenol, given intravenously or sublingually, is useful in a chronically slow sinus rate. In an acute situation, 1 mg of isoproterenol may be dissolved in 500 ml of solution and the rate of drip monitored by the patient's response. CAUTION: Isoproterenol in the presence of acute myocardial infarction is a two-edged sword—while the drug speeds the heart rate, it also exacts a payment in the form of increased oxygen requirements by the myocardium. When myocardial blood flow has been compromised, this may be a very dangerous demand and may be one that the coronary blood flow cannot meet. Studies with experimentally produced infarcts have shown that isoproterenol actually increases the size of the infarct by imposing too great an oxygen demand on marginally perfused myocardial tissues. In the presence of infarction, therefore, atrial pacing is safer and is probably more effective and reliable than isoproterenol.

Failure of conduction from atria to ventricles. When the A-V node is diseased, escape rhythms will appear simply because the S-A impulse does not penetrate the A-V node to the ventricles or penetrates it only occasionally. In such patients, the appearance of an escape ectopic rhythm is almost always a lifesaving phenomenon. Therapy is directed toward accelerating conduction through the A-V node by removing toxic effects (digitalis, quinidine, or elevated potassium) or by use of atropine and isoproterenol.

When the A-V node does not function at all—that is, when complete heart block is present—the junctional or ventricular rhythms driving the heart are lifesaving. If the rate of discharge of such a rhythm is inadequate, ventricular pacing should be used to produce a rate consistent with optimal cardiac performance.

Atrial pacing. Transvenous atrial and ventricular pacing are described in Chapter 20. Any physician who cares for cardiac patients should be able to carry out this simple bedside procedure. If a S-A node does not respond to drug stimulation, atrial pacing should be used to provide a normal rate of stimulation for the heartbeat. This is particularly important in patients with myocardial infarction with inadequate cardiac output who may be in shock or in a state of heart failure. Atrial pacing is a particularly useful mode of treatment since it provides a normal sequence of atrial and ventricular contraction, thus ensuring maximum cardiac output per beat. The atrial rate is set to exceed the rate of the ectopic pacemaker by a sufficient margin to suppress ectopic pacemaker.

Idionodal and idioventricular rhythms and cardiac output

Escape ectopic rhythms are frequently lifesaving, but they are not completely innocuous. Sometimes an ectopic ventricular or junctional pacemaker will begin firing very close to the rate of the S-A node (Fig. 5-13). This is quite likely to happen after myocardial infarction. It is commonly stated that such escape rhythms are harmless, but this is not always true.

When atrial synchronization is not present—when atrial contraction does not precede ventricular contraction by a normal interval—cardiac output falls significantly because of the lack of atrial "kick." The physician will remember that atrial systole forces a residue of blood into the ventricles and "supercharges" the ventricles just prior to ventricular systole. This atrial "kick" has been shown in recent years to be very important in sustaining cardiac output. When some degree of heart damage is present, withdrawal of this atrial effect may result in a fall of as much as 25% in cardiac output. While a healthy individual can sustain the loss of atrial synchronization without significant untoward effect, the patient who has suffered a myocardial infarct with a fall in output to marginal levels simply cannot afford the further drop that comes from a loss of normal atrial synchronization. When a patient in the acute stage of myocardial infarction goes into a sustained idioventricular rhythm, the blood pressure will often be noted to drop significantly, and, in some cases, symptoms of shock or failure may appear. In these patients, restoration of a normal synchronized beat may be lifesaving. It is therefore imperative to restore a normal atrial-ventricular synchronized rhythm, either by speeding the S-A node with atropine or by atrial pacing.

Despite statements in medical literature to the contrary, an idioventricular or idionodal rhythm appearing in a patient with severely compromised cardiac function may threaten life. Every effort should be made to restore an atrial rhythm, by acceleration of the S-A node or by pacing from the atrium.

REFERENCES

Gianelly, R., and others: Effect of lidocaine on ventricular arrhythmias in patients with coronary heart disease, New Eng. J. Med. **277**:1215-1219, 1967.

Konecke, L. L., and Knoebel, S.: Nonparoxysmal junctional tachycardia complicating acute myocardial infarction, Circulation **45**:367-374, 1972.

Marriott, H. J. L., and Menendez, M.: A-V dissociation revisited, Progr. Cardiovasc. Dis. **8**:522-538, 1966.

Mogensen, L.: Ventricular tachyarrhythmias and lignocaine prophylaxis in acute myocardial infarction: a clinical and therapeutic study, Acta Med. Scand. (Suppl.), p. 513, 1970.

Moss, A., and others: Ventricular arrhythmias 3 weeks after acute myocardial infarction, Ann. Intern. Med. **75**:837-841, 1971.

Roelandt, J., and Schamroth, L.: Parasystolic ventricular tachycardia: observations on differential stimulus threshold as possible mechanism for exit block, Brit. Heart J. **33**:505-512, 1971.

Schamroth, L.: Idioventricular tachycardia, J. Electrocardiol. **1**:205-212, 1968.

Zipes, D. S., and Fisch, C.: Accelerated ventricular rhythm, Arch. Intern. Med. **129**:650-652, 1972.

6 Ventricular aberration and ventricular fusion

So far, all discussions in this book have assumed that a beat arising in the atria or in the A-V junction is conducted normally down through the ventricular conducting network. This is not always true. This chapter will describe two variations of conduction through the ventricular network that the student must learn to recognize and to use.

ABERRATION

Aberrant conduction means that some part of the ventricular conducting network is transmitting the exciting impulse very slowly or not transmitting it at all. Abnormally slow conduction takes place because some part of the ventricular conducting network is still in its relative refractory state when the next depolarizing or exciting wave arrives. Complete failure of conduction in some part of the ventricular conducting network will result when the exciting wave finds the ventricular conducting tissue still in its absolute refractory state—that is, not capable of conducting at all.

The QRS complex produced by aberrant conduction will always differ from the QRS produced when the ventricular conducting tissues are functioning normally. The aberrant QRS will always have a different shape than the normal QRS, and it will usually be wider (Fig. 6-1). In simple terms, picture the ventricular conducting tissues as a network of blacktop roads down which the exciting impulse can move swiftly under normal circumstances. Picture further an area of the blacktop road torn up and converted into a rutted lane, so that the exciting wave must move over it very slowly. Picture another area of the road completely blocked off, so that the exciting wave must detour around the diseased area. These basic phenomena of slowing and detouring really describe aberration, although the electrophysics can become exceedingly complicated when examined in detail.

The most extreme form of aberrant intraventricular conduction is complete bundle branch block. The term "bundle branch block" means that one of the two bundle branches is completely blocked—it is completely incapable of conducting an impulse. The block must lie somewhere near the origin of the bundle before it breaks up into smaller branches.

When one bundle branch is blocked, the exciting wave moves quickly down the normal bundle branch, inscribing the first part of the ventricular complex, and then enters the "blocked" side of the heart by a backward route around the apex and up through the myocardium, which is always a slow process. This slow conduction is the key to the diagnosis of bundle branch block. *When either bundle branch is com-*

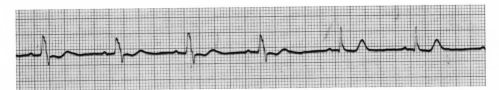

Fig. 6-1. Aberrant conduction. Note that the first four ventricular complexes on this strip are wide and have a different configuration from the last four normally conducted narrow QRS complexes on the right. This tracing illustrates both features of ventricular aberration—abnormally slow conduction within the ventricles, producing widening of the QRS, and an abnormal course of conduction within the ventricles, producing a different configuration of QRS when compared to normally conducted beats.

pletely blocked, the QRS complex will always be at least .12 second wide; it may be wider, it will never be less. A QRS complex .12 second in duration, therefore, means one of two things: either the beat arises from a ventricular ectopic focus or complete bundle branch block is present.

Differential diagnosis between ventricular ectopic beats and bundle branch block. To differentiate between a sinus or ectopic atrial beat with bundle branch block, *the P wave makes the difference!* When you see a wide QRS (.12 second or more), see if it is preceded at a normal conducting distance by a P wave. If it is, the diagnosis is bundle branch block. A wide QRS complex *not* preceded at a normal conducting distance by a P wave is a ventricular ectopic beat.

Impossible differentiation. Remember that junctional beats often have no visible P wave; *therefore, a QRS complex .12 second wide may be a ventricular ectopic beat or a junctional ectopic beat in the presence of bundle branch block. Either kind of beat produces a wide QRS without a P wave: it is often impossible to tell them apart.* (Fusion beats, described later in this chapter, sometimes provide the clue that makes this differentiation possible.)

Distinguishing left and right bundle branch block. The configuration of lead V_1 makes the distinction between left and right bundle branch block a simple matter most of the time. Follow these simple steps in recognition:

1. Lead V_1 normally consists of a small R followed by a deep S.
2. If lead V_1 has a normal configuration and if the ventricular complex is .12 second wide, *left* bundle branch block is present (Fig. 6-2, *A*).
3. If lead V_1 is "upside down" with a tall, terminal R wave instead of an S and if the QRS complex is .12 second wide, *right* bundle branch block is present (Fig. 6-2, *B*).

As a further confirmation, remember that leads V_6 and I are electrically "opposite" from V_1. Therefore, in the two varieties of bundle branch block, these leads will have an opposite or "upside down" configuration from V_1 (Fig. 6-2).

Less severe forms of aberration will produce a QRS complex less than .12 second wide, almost always with a different shape than the normal QRS (Fig. 6-1). At such times, some of the smaller branches or fascicles of the bundle branch system are functioning slowly or not at all. In recent years electrocardiographers have learned to recognize several specific patterns of aberrant conduction localized to specific subdivisions of the main bundle branches. These are described in Chapter 8.

At this time the student need remember only that (1) aberrant conduction within the ventricular conducting system is common, (2) it may appear in a specific pattern of left or right bundle branch block, or (3) it may appear as a nonspecific widening and deformity of the QRS complex, indicating delayed, "roundabout" conduction.

FUSION

In all examples shown so far in this book, the ventricles have been activated from a single source; they have been activated by a wave entering from above, down

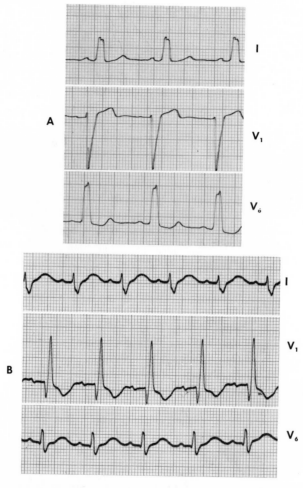

Fig. 6-2. A, Left bundle branch block. Note that the QRS configuration in V_1 is normal, except for the widening of the S wave. An rS in lead V_1 with a wide S wave, bringing the QRS to a total duration of .12 second, makes the diagnosis of left bundle branch block. Note that leads I and V_6 look alike; this is because they are both recording from the left side of the electric field of the heart. Note, too, that the QRS in both these leads is "opposite" in configuration from V_1. **B,** Right bundle branch block. Note that V_1 is now "upside down" with a wide tall terminal R wave instead of the terminal S wave noted in left bundle branch block. Again, note that leads I and V_6 look alike and are basically opposite in configuration from V_1.

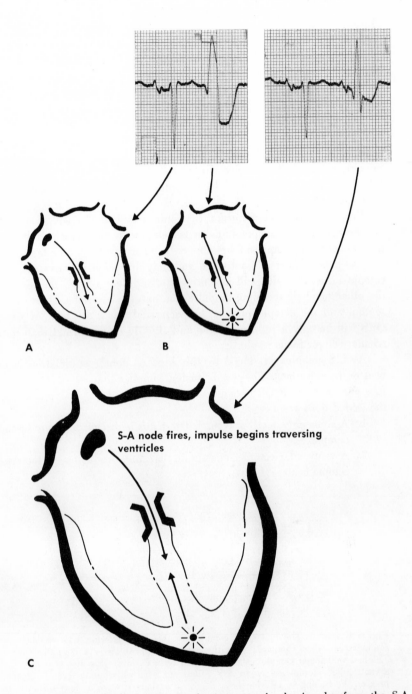

Fig. 6-3. Somewhere in the ventricular conducting network, the impulse from the S-A node collides with the impulse from the ventricular focus. The ventricles are stimulated from two directions and a fused QRS is the result. Fused QRS complexes are intermediate in form between normal and PVC; a P wave precedes the QRS at a short interval.

through the normal conducting system, or they have been activated "from below" by a ventricular ectopic beat.

Sometimes the ventricles are activated from two sources or directions at once (Fig. 6-3). Imagine that a wave moving down the normal conducting system from the S-A node has penetrated a third of the way across the ventricles, beginning ventricular action. Suppose that at this precise time a ventricular ectopic focus fires, activating the lower part of the ventricles while the S-A node is activating the upper portion. The two activating waves will collide somewhere in the ventricles, and the chambers will thus have been stimulated from two directions at once.

The QRS complex produced by such dual stimualtion will be a hybrid—it will be a cross between the grossly abnormal QRS that would have been produced by the ventricular ectopic focus and the normal QRS that would have resulted had the sinus impulse activated the ventricles completely. This fused QRS will not be as wide as the full-blown ventricular ectopic beat would have been, but it will be wider than the normal complex.

How wide and *how abnormal* the ventricular complex will be will depend on how far the ventricular ectopic impulse travels across the ventricles before it meets the normal activating impulse from above. In other words, if nine tenths of the total ventricular mass is normally activated and only one tenth is activated by the ventricular ectopic focus, the QRS will be only slightly different from the normal complex. On the other hand, if the sinus impulse has only penetrated a short distance down the septum and the ectopic impulse has activated the great bulk of the ventricles, the QRS will be only a little narrower and slightly more normal than a full-blown ventricular ectopic focus would be.

A QRS complex produced by this kind of double stimulation is called a fusion beat or Dressler beat. The word "fusion" implies that two different activating waves fuse to form a single QRS complex. One can be sure that fusion is taking place only if these conditions are met:

1. A sinus or other supraventricular focus is discharging, producing normal QRS complexes.

2. A ventricular ectopic focus is discharging, producing characteristic ventricular ectopic beats.

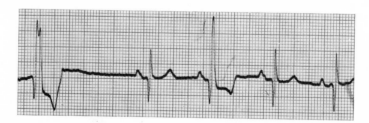

Fig. 6-4. Fusion. The first QRS complex in this strip is wide (.14 second) and has a bizarre configuration when compared with the second beat, which is a normally conducted sinus beat. The first ventricular complex is not preceded by a P wave; this first beat may therefore be either a ventricular ectopic beat or an A-V junctional beat with bundle branch block. The third complex on the tracing is a fusion beat. There is a sinus P wave a short distance ahead of it (note that the P-R is shorter than in the preceding normally conducted beat), and the QRS complex is "intermediate" in form between the sinus beats and the wide ectopic beat which begins the strip. The presence of a fusion beat identifies the first beat in this tracing as a ventricular ectopic beat.

3. One or more beats are seen in the record with an abnormally *short* P-R interval and a QRS complex with a shape "somewhere in between" the shape of a normal beat and a ventricular ectopic beat (Fig. 6-4).

This "hybrid" QRS complex must come *just after* a P wave—fusion can take place only if an atrial complex has started to penetrate the ventricles from above, just before the ventricular ectopic focus fires; hence, logic dictates that a P wave must precede the fused QRS complex by a short distance.

Significance of fusion beats. Fusion beats provide a solution to a diagnostic dilemma described earlier in this chapter. Remember that an A-V junctional beat with bundle branch block will look exactly like a ventricular ectopic beat. Sometimes it is very important to distinguish between the two types of beat for therapeutic or prognostic purposes. *If fusion beats are detected in the tracing, it establishes the fact that the wide QRS complexes are, in fact, ventricular ectopic beats, since a "fused" QRS complex can result only from the meeting of a ventricular ectopic beat with an impulse penetrating the ventricles from above.* To put it another way, the phenomenon of fusion means that two impulses are meeting somewhere in the ventricular conducting network; this can happen only if one of the impulses arises within the ventricles while the other penetrates from above.

Fusion beats will be included in tracings from this point on, as will aberrantly conducted beats. The student should be ready to recognize both phenomena, since they are of great practical importance.

7 Problems, practice, and reinforcement: 1

At this point, the student should have acquired certain skills; specifically, he should be able to (1) distinguish normal from abnormal atrioventricular and intraventricular conduction (the student should know the limits of normal for the P-R interval and for the duration of the QRS complex); (2) recognize sinus rhythms; (3) recognize sites of origin of ectopic beats; (4) distinguish premature from escape firing; (5) distinguish left from right bundle branch block; and (6) recognize ventricular fusion and aberration.

It is now time to use these skills in solving practical clinical problems. Answer the specific questions regarding each problem strip and then compare your answers with the correct answers.

PROBLEM 1: This rhythm is noted on the oscilloscope of a patient in the acute stage of a myocardial infarction (Fig. 7-1).

QUESTIONS:

1. Basic rhythm?
2. Source of fourth beat in upper strip?
3. Source of next to last beat on lower strip?
4. Relation of these two beats?
5. Treatment?

ANSWERS:

1. The basic rhythm is a normal sinus rhythm.
2. The fourth beat, upper strip, is wide (.12 second) and is *not* preceded at a conducting distance by a P wave. Conclusion: This is a possible ventricular ectopic beat.
3. In the next to last beat, bottom strip, the P wave comes just ahead of the QRS complex, too close for normal A-V conduction. The QRS complex is "intermediate" in shape between the normal sinus complexes and the ectopic beat in the top strip. Conclusion: *Fusion* is apparent in this beat, the P wave having partially penetrated the ventricles just before the ventricular focus fired.
4. Presence of a fusion beat identifies the ectopic beat in the top strip as being definitely ventricular in orgin.
5. If ventricular premature contractions appear frequently, suppressive drugs may be indicated, for example, lidocaine, quinidine, or procainamide.

PROBLEM 2: A patient with a history of arteriosclerotic heart disease and recurrent angina pectoris manifests these changes while a routine electrocardiogram is being recorded (Fig. 7-2).

QUESTIONS:
1. Basic rhythm?
2. Reason for change in QRS configuration between left and right side of strips?
3. Significance?

ANSWERS:
1. This is a normal sinus rhythm.
2. The wide QRS complexes on the left represent aberrant intraventricular conduction associated with a slightly more rapid sinus rate than on the right, where intraventricular conduction is normal. Appearance of aberrant conduction at the more rapid rate means that some part of the ventricular conducting system has a prolonged refractory period and can conduct normally only up to a certain rate. Above that rate, the area in question fails to conduct or conducts slowly, producing the wide ventricular complexes on the left.
3. The presence of *rate-dependent aberration* as illustrated here implies organic disease or toxic effect within the ventricular conducting system.

PROBLEM 3: A patient is seen in the emergency room describing "rapid pounding" of the heart and a sense of weakness. The disorder appeared abruptly during normal activity (Fig. 7-3).

QUESTIONS:
1. Diagnosis of rhythm?
2. Significance?
3. Therapy?

ANSWERS:
1. The rate is rapid (150) and the rhythm is perfectly regular. There are no

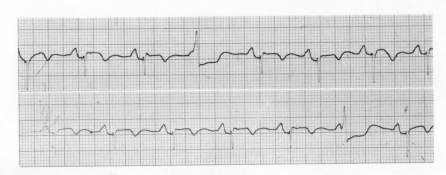

Fig. 7-1. Problem 1.

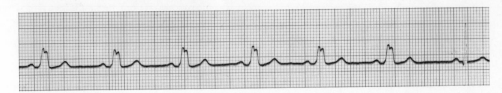

Fig. 7-2. Problem 2.

visible P waves; the ventricular complexes are wide (.12 second). Presumptive diagnosis is therefore paroxysmal ventricular tachycardia. (Other possible diagnosis is A-V junctional tachycardia with bundle branch block.)

2. The prognosis is always serious—ventricular tachycardia almost always implies significant organic heart disease.
3. Suppressive drugs (lidocaine, procainamide, quinidine) or electroversion may be used.

PROBLEM 4: The rhythm illustrated appears in the tracing of a patient in the coronary care unit with a diagnosis of myocardial infarction and probable congestive heart failure (Fig. 7-4).

QUESTIONS:
1. Type of arrhythmia?
2. Proof of origin of rhythm?
3. Significance?
4. Treatment?

ANSWERS:
1. The first four complexes are wide (.14 second) and are not preceded by P waves. The rate is in the normal range (71). Presumptive diagnosis is therefore idioventricular rhythm or accelerated idioventricular rhythm. Normal sinus rhythm is seen in the center of the strip, and a ventricular pacemaker resumes firing on the right.
2. A slight degree of fusion is visible in the fourth beat; obvious fusion is seen in the next to last beat. Fusion beats identify the ectopic pacemaker as being indisputably in the ventricle.
3. This kind of rhythm becomes serious when cardiac output is compromised. In a diseased heart the cardiac output will fall about 25% during the ectopic rhythm because of lack of atrial "kick." In the case described here, therefore,

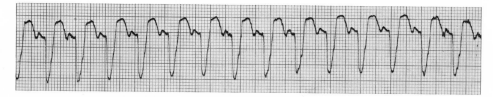

Fig. 7-3. Problem 3.

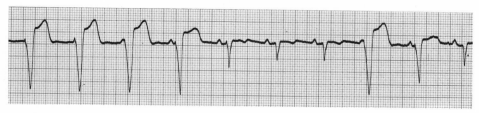

Fig. 7-4. Problem 4.

this rhythm is indeed significant and restoration of normal sinus rhythm is important.

4. Since this is an idioventricular rhythm and *not* a ventricular tachycardia, suppressive drugs are not used. Therapy is instead directed at acceleration of the S-A node with atropine or by pacing.

PROBLEM 5: This rhythm is detected in a 25-year-old female who enters the emergency room complaining of faintness and nervousness that appeared abruptly while she was walking down the street (Fig. 7-5).

QUESTIONS:

1. Basic rhythm?
2. Significance?

ANSWERS:

1. The rate is rapid (260) and the rhythm is perfectly regular. Paroxysmal tachycardia is therefore the presumptive diagnosis. The QRS complexes are narrow (.06 second). The ectopic focus must lie in the upper portion of the heart, the atria or the A-V junction. Because of the rapid rate it is not possible to be sure whether P waves are hidden in T waves or not. The diagnosis, therefore, is *paroxysmal supraventricular tachycardia*.

2. Supraventricular tachycardia is not necessarily serious and it may occur in the absence of any heart disease. Treatment may include carotid sinus stimulation, digitalis, quinidine, or sympathomimetic drugs.

PROBLEM 6: This tracing is recorded in a healthy patient who is free of symptoms and who is having an annual complete physical examination (Fig. 7-6).

QUESTIONS:

1. Abnormality of rhythm?
2. Significance?

ANSWERS:

1. Normal sinus rhythm is present throughout, except for the fifth beat. This

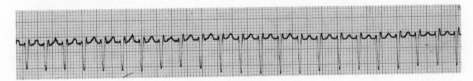

Fig. 7-5. Problem 5.

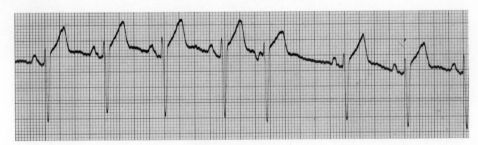

Fig. 7-6. Problem 6.

beat is premature and therefore ectopic. The QRS is like the QRS complex of the sinus beats; therefore, the ectopic beat must be supraventricular in origin. An abnormally shaped P wave precedes the QRS complex by .13 second. Conclusion: The ectopic beat is atrial in origin.

2. Occasional atrial premature beats have no significance and they do not imply heart disease.

PROBLEM 7: A patient in the coronary care unit 4 days after a myocardial infarct describes pounding and thumping of his heart (Fig. 7-7).

QUESTIONS:

1. Type of rhythm?
2. Proof?
3. Significance?
4. Treatment?

ANSWERS:

1. The diagnosis is normal sinus rhythm with short runs of paroxysmal ventricular tachycardia. The first beat is a normal sinus beat; it is followed by a run of wide beats without P waves appearing rapidly and regularly. (Ignore standardizing signal in the fourth beat.) Presumptive diagnosis is paroxysmal ventricular tachycardia.

2. To be sure that the wide beats really come from a ventricular focus, look through the rest of the strip for fusion beats. Note the third beat from the right-hand side. This beat has a short P-R interval with a QRS complex wider than the sinus beats and narrower than the full-blown ventricular ectopic beats. The conclusion is that this is a fusion beat, which again identifies the ectopic pacemaker as ventricular.

3. In a patient with an acute myocardial infarct, this is a very dangerous arrhythmia; it may precede ventricular fibrillation.

4. Suppressive therapy with lidocaine, procainamide, or quinidine is indicated.

PROBLEM 8: A patient in the coronary care unit in congestive heart failure who is taking digoxin, 0.25 mg twice a day, manifests this arrhythmia (Fig. 7-8).

QUESTIONS:

1. Type of rhythm?

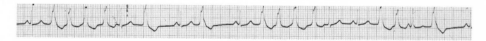

Fig. 7-7. Problem 7.

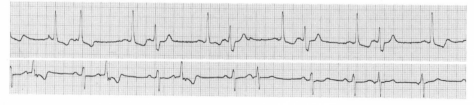

Fig. 7-8. Problem 8.

2. Proof?
3. Significance?
4. Treatment?

ANSWERS:

1. A sinus rhythm interrupted by an ectopic beat that appears every other beat is present throughout most of the tracing (pulsus bigeminus). The first ectopic beat (third beat on the tracing) has a QRS complex exactly like the sinus beat. This beat is therefore supraventricular in origin, that is, it may arise in the atria or the A-V junction. There seems to be a small, inverted P wave a short distance before the ectopic beat, but the exact P-R interval cannot be determined because the P wave is buried in the preceding T wave. The remainder of the premature beats in the top strip appear at almost the same interval after the sinus beat and are all preceded by the same small atrial complex. The QRS complex in each of these ectopic beats, however, is wide.

2. *Problem in reasoning:* Is the widened QRS complex of these premature beats caused by aberrant conduction from a supraventricular complex, or are these ventricular ectopic beats? *Solution:* Measure very carefully from the sinus beats to the ectopic beats and notice that the wide QRS complexes are definitely closer to the preceding sinus beat than is the normally conducted ectopic beat on the left-hand side of the strip (.28 second versus .35 second). *Conclusion:* The ectopic beats coming close after the preceding sinus beat are appearing "too early" for normal conduction through the ventricles; hence, they are being conducted aberrantly. Those beats appearing slightly later find the ventricular conducting tissues out of the refractory state and ready to conduct. *Further conclusion:* The refractory period of some part of the ventricular conducting tissues is abnormally prolonged, implying intrinsic disease or toxicity.

    Second exercise in reasoning: Are the ectopic beats atrial or junctional? Look at the last beat in the bottom strip. Here the ectopic focus has fired as a "postmature" or escape beat. Note the small inverted P wave .09 second before the QRS complex. *Conclusion:* The ectopic focus is in the A-V junction, since this P-R interval is too short for conduction from the atria.

    Full diagnosis: Pulsus bigeminus, produced by ectopic focus in the A-V junction, with aberrant conduction of many of the premature beats is the diagnosis.

3. Repetitive A-V junctional firing is a common manifestation of digitalis toxicity.

4. Discontinue digitalis and observe for change in rhythm.

PROBLEM 9: An exercise in reasoning! A patient seen 2 days following myocardial infarction manifests the rhythm in the top strip (Fig. 7-9).

QUESTIONS:

1. Origin of rhythm?
2. Significance?
3. Treatment?

ANSWERS:

1. The basic rhythm consists of wide QRS complexes without P waves; the rate is 58. Two premature beats with wider QRS complexes and no P waves interrupt this basic rhythm. Possibilities include idioventricular rhythm inter-

rupted by two premature ventricular beats, or A-V junctional rhythm with bundle branch block interrupted by two premature ventricular beats. Look at the left-hand side of the bottom strip for the answer. Normal sinus rhythm appears, with a P-R interval of .16 second. *QRS complexes during sinus rhythm look exactly like the QRS complexes in the dominant rhythm in the top strip.*

Conclusion: The wide QRS complexes in the top strip must represent A-V junctional beats with bundle branch block, since the course of the activating wave across the ventricles is clearly the same in the sinus beats in the bottom strip and in the unidentified regular rhythm in the top strip.

Further observation: The sinus rhythm ends with a ventricular premature beat and the junctional rhythm resumes. Note the small retrograde P wave in the T wave of the ventricular premature beat. Obviously the atria have been fired in retrograde fashion by the impulse coming up from the ventricular ectopic focus. In the pause following this premature discharge of the atria, the A-V junctional pacemaker "escapes" and sets the rhythm. Note further that all ventricular ectopic beats in this strip show small retrograde P waves on the upslope of the T. It is likely that the S-A node is being suppressed by continued retrograde firing from the ventricular ectopic beats. This recurrent suppression allows the A-V junction to escape and to set the rhythm.

2. Junctional rhythm is an inefficient rhythm in terms of cardiac output. In a critically ill patient restoration of sinus rhythm may be crucial.

3. Accelerate the S-A node with atropine or with atrial pacing. If ventricular premature beats persist after S-A acceleration, treat the ventricular ectopic beats with suppressive drugs.

PROBLEM 10: Lead V_1 is recorded in two patients (Fig. 7-10).

QUESTION: Diagnoses?

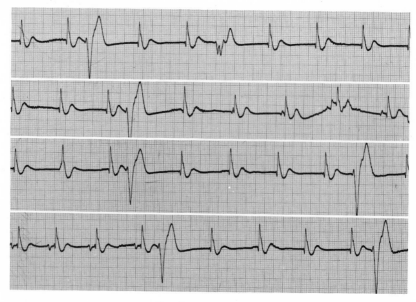

Fig. 7-9. Problem 9.

ANSWER: Diagnoses are left bundle branch block and right bundle branch block. If there is any doubt about these diagnoses, go back to Chapter 6 and reread carefully.

PROBLEM 11: Another exercise in reasoning: The slow rhythm illustrated here appears in a patient the day following a myocardial infarction (Fig. 7-11).

QUESTIONS:
1. Reason for irregular rhythm?
2. Reason for pause in the center of the strip? Is the A-V node functioning normally or is it occasionally failing to conduct?
3. What measures should be taken?

ANSWERS:
1. The first two beats reveal a normal sinus rhythm with a slow rate (50); sinus bradycardia is therefore present. The third beat is premature. The QRS is similar to that of the sinus beats, although it is smaller in amplitude. This beat is not preceded by a P wave and is therefore a premature A-V junctional beat. A P wave follows the premature beat; this P wave "measures out" exactly with the P waves of the sinus beats. Conclusion: The second visible P wave is a sinus P wave that has no connection with the preceding premature beat.
2. There is a pause following the second visible sinus P wave ended by another QRS complex with a different configuration than that of the first three. This QRS complex is .12 second wide. Two possibilities exist: either this is a ventricular ectopic beat or it is an aberrantly conducted beat from the third sinus

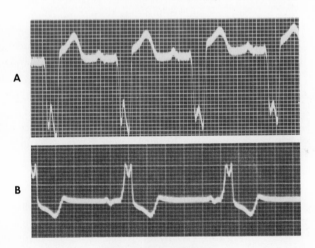

Fig. 7-10. Problem 10.

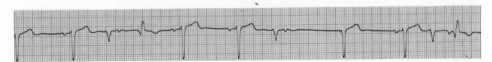

Fig. 7-11. Problem 11.

P wave, with a very long P-R interval. This cannot be decided yet—hold the question in abeyance until the rest of the strip has been analyzed!

The fifth and sixth are normal sinus beats, followed again, in the seventh beat, by another A-V junctional premature beat exactly like the third beat. Again, the sinus P wave comes at its normal interval following the A-V junctional beat and this time the sinus P wave is completely blocked—that is, it is not conducted to the ventricles. The eighth beat consists of a normal QRS complex with a P wave immediately in front of it. This P-R interval is too short for A-V conduction to take place, and the conclusion is that a sinus P wave has simply "run into" a junctional beat, or, to put it another way, a sinus P wave and a junctional escape beat are partially superimposed. The ninth beat is a normal sinus beat, followed again by an A-V junctional beat, which in turn is followed by a sinus P wave. This time the sinus P wave is followed at a very short interval by a wide QRS complex that looks exactly like the fourth ventricular complex. Conclusion: The eleventh beat and the fourth beat must represent ventricular ectopic beats, since the eleventh QRS complex comes much too close to the P wave for A-V conduction to have taken place.

Final diagnosis: Diagnosis is sinus bradycardia, occasional A-V junctional premature beats, and nonconducted sinus P waves because of refractoriness in the A-V node produced by the A-V junctional premature beats and occasional ventricular ectopic beats. Conclusions: The A-V node is capable of functioning; the reason for nonconduction of the third and sixth sinus P waves is simply *interference* by the junctional beats that discharge just before the sinus P waves. The reason for nonconduction of the next-to-last sinus P wave is the coincidental firing of a ventricular ectopic focus just after the P wave, before the sinus impulse has time to be conducted to the ventricles.

3. The basic problem is a slow discharge of the S-A node; therefore, the use of atropine is indicated. A more rapid sinus rate would probably suppress the junctional ectopic beats, as well as the ventricular ectopic beats, by simply "overdriving." Long pauses, like the pause in the center of this strip, are always hazardous in a patient after a myocardial infarct and should be eradicated whenever possible.

NOTE: The concept of *interference* is introduced in this tracing. Look carefully at the eighth beat. A sinus P wave is present, but about halfway through the P wave a QRS complex is inscribed. Clearly, just as the atrial wave was approaching the A-V nodal junction, an ectopic pacemaker in the junctional tissue discharged and the sinus impulse could proceed no further. Thus there is failure of transmission of the activating wave from atria to ventricles because of the interference of the ectopic pacemaker. *"Interference," in terms of cardiac arrhythmias, simply means failure of propagation of an impulse because of a refractory state in the conducting tissues produced by discharge of another pacemaker.* When an ectopic pacemaker discharges in such a way as to prevent propagation of a sinus impulse, the ectopic pacemaker is called the "interfering" pacemaker. The sinus P wave following the seventh beat is not transmitted to the ventricles because of interference by the preceding A-V junctional beat that has left the A-V nodal tissues refractory.

8 Atrioventricular block

The A-V conducting system consists of the A-V node, the bundle of His, and the upper or proximal portions of the bundle branches. Disease or toxic dysfunction of any part of these conducting tissues may produce *delay in transmission* or *failure of transmission* of the exciting impulse from the atria to the ventricles. This kind of delay or failure in transmission is termed atrioventricular (A-V) block.

CLASSIFICATION

To classify A-V block, the physician asks two questions:
1. Where is the block? (Is the block localized in the A-V node or in the proximal portions of the bundle branch system?)
2. How severe is the block? (Is there simple delay in transmission from atria to ventricles? Is there *occasional* failure of transmission from the atria to ventricles? Is there *complete* failure of transmission from atria to ventricles?)

ANATOMIC SITE (Fig. 8-1)

A-V block will be localized in one of two areas—the A-V node proper or the upper bundle branch system. Block may take place within the bundle of His, but it is almost impossible to document this accurately.

Electrocardiographers for years suspected that A-V block was often caused by delay or failure of transmission in the upper bundle branch system, but it was not until catheter techniques of study were developed that it was possible to prove this. Remember that passage of the activating wave through the A-V node and bundle of His is electrically "silent"—no deflection is produced at the surface of the body in the conventional electrocardiogram during this passage. When a catheter is suitably placed inside the heart, however, it is possible to record the activation of the bundle of His; this produces a characteristic short spike referred to as the "H" deflection or spike. Using this type of catheter recording, it is possible to divide A-V conduction into three components:
1. The interval from discharge of the S-A node to arrival of the activating wave at the A-V node. This is measured simply by the width of the P wave.
2. Passage through the A-V node. This is the interval from the end of atrial passage to the beginning of activation of the bundle of His, as detected by the His deflection on the catheter-recorded electrogram.
3. The interval from activation of the bundle of His to completion of activation of the ventricles

For convenience, the first two categories of conduction are usually lumped together, and block in the A-V node is referred to as atrial-His block or A-H block. Block below the bundle of His, presumably in the upper bundle branch system, is referred to as His-Purkinje or His-ventricular block. The abbreviations H-P and H-V are used to describe this part of conduction.

His-Purkinje block is generally much more serious than atrial-His (A-V nodal) block. Differentiating between the two sites of block, therefore, may be of profound therapeutic and prognostic significance.

It is clearly not practical to catheterize every case of A-V block, nor is it necessary. By analyzing the *functional degree* of block and by detecting certain specific combinations of delayed conduction, the physician can arrive at an approximate localization of block and can make some sound prognostic and therapeutic deductions. In this chapter, therefore, the functional types or degrees of block will be outlined in detail and later will be correlated with the anatomic sites of block.

FUNCTIONAL CLASSIFICATION

A-V block is divided into three types or degrees of block:
1. First-degree block, or block in which all sinus impulses reach the ventricles. The sinus impulses take a longer time than normal in the passage from atria to ventricles.
2. Second-degree block, or block in which *some* of the sinus impulses reach the ventricles while others are blocked in the A-V conducting system. There are several subtypes of second-degree block.
3. Third-degree block, block in which *none* of the sinus impulses reaches the ventricles. There is complete failure of transmission of the A-V conducting tissues.

First-degree block

The P-R interval is prolonged (longer than .20 second) in the adult. There is one P wave for each ventricular complex. The P-R interval is constant. The tracing

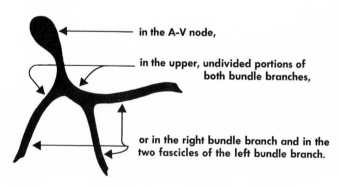

Delayed conduction or failure of conduction from atria to ventricles may be the result of disease or dysfunction in one of three sites:

in the A-V node,

in the upper, undivided portions of both bundle branches,

or in the right bundle branch and in the two fascicles of the left bundle branch.

Fig. 8-1. Possible sites of A-V block.

will look exactly like a sinus mechanism except for the prolonged P-R interval
(Fig. 8-2).

The tracing shown in Fig. 8-3 illustrates first-degree A-V block. Note that the
P-R interval is about .36 second.

Any P-R interval longer than .20 second should be regarded as abnormal. In

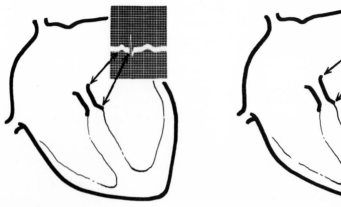

Normal conduction does not take
longer than .20 second

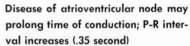

Disease of atrioventricular node may
prolong time of conduction; P-R interval increases (.35 second)

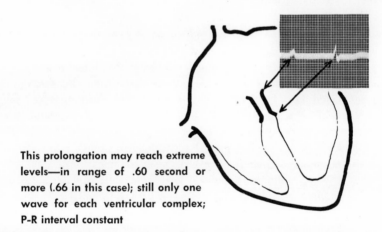

This prolongation may reach extreme
levels—in range of .60 second or
more (.66 in this case); still only one
wave for each ventricular complex;
P-R interval constant

Fig. 8-2. Partial A-V block (first-degree block). In this type of block, each impulse from the
sinus node is conducted to the ventricles. Because of disease in the A-V node, the impulse takes
a longer time than normal in its passage through the node. The P-R interval is constant.

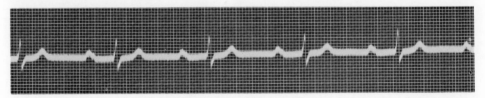

Fig. 8-3. First-degree A-V block.

exceptional circumstances transient prolongation may be seen in healthy persons, changing with posture, breathing, and so on. Usually, however, prolongation of the P-R interval above .20 second indicates pathology.

In children the P-R interval is shorter. Normal values for children under 5 years of age range up to .16 second, and for children from 6 to 13 years of age .18 second is probably the upper limit of normal. These figures are very important clinically, since A-V block will be encountered in children in the course of various acute myocardial infections and inflammations—diphtheritic, viral, rheumatic, and so on. P-R prolongation can reach fantastic proportions. Values of almost a full second have been recorded, and figures from .60 to .70 second are not rare.

Second-degree block

REMEMBER: Second-degree block is that kind of block in which some sinus impulses reach the ventricles while others do not. There are three main types of second-degree block:

1. Fixed ratio/fixed P-R interval
2. Changing P-R (Wenckebach phenomenon)
3. Occasional blocked P waves, or Mobitz Type 2 block

Fixed ratio/fixed P-R interval

This may seem a clumsy title, but nobody has yet proposed a really good name for this type of second-degree block. Figs. 8-4 and 8-5 illustrate this phenomenon. Note that the P waves appear at regular intervals, but note further that every other one is blocked. This is therefore called 2:1 block. *Inspect the P-R intervals of the conducted beats. Note that they are all the same.* This is the diagnostic feature of this type of block. The ratio may be anything from 2:1 to 8:1, but the beats conducted through the A-V node will show a constant P-R interval as long as the ratio of conduction remains the same. If the ratio of conduction changes, the P-R interval of the conducted beats will change. For any given ratio of atrial to ventricular beats, there will be a constant P-R interval for the beats reaching the ventricles. Examples of 2:1 block are shown in Figs. 8-6 and 8-7. Note that the P-R intervals of the conducted beats may be normal or prolonged, *but they are always the same.*

Sometimes the ratio changes. The block may change from 2:1 to 4:1 for several beats, then to 6:1, and finally back to 2:1. This will produce a grossly irregular pulse. Such changes in ratio are illustrated in Figs. 8-8 and 8-9. In Fig. 8-8 the first two sinus impulses are conducted to the ventricles, while the third is blocked. Thus, there is a ratio of three P waves to two QRS complexes: 3:2 block is present. A 2:1 block is present throughout the rest of the strip. The same shift in degree of block is present in Fig. 8-9. Note that a 3:2 block produces a pulsus bigeminus or paired ventricular pulse. At the bedside, the impression would be that a premature beat was occurring every other beat, which is the usual cause of pulsus bigeminus. Of course, nothing of the sort is really happening, but only an electrocardiogram can make this clear.

Changing P-R or Wenckebach phenomenon

The Wenckebach phenomenon produces a much more common form of second-degree block than the fixed P-R type. The Wenckebach phenomenon is illustrated in Fig. 8-10.

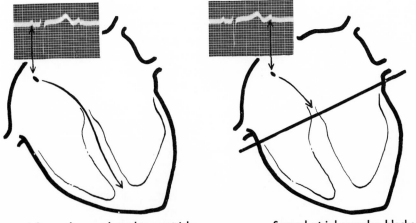

First atrial complex conducted to ventricles   Second atrial complex blocked

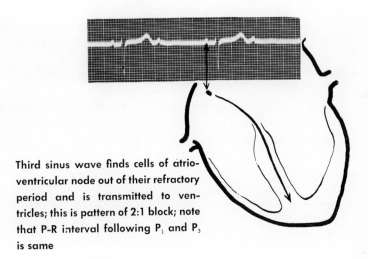

Third sinus wave finds cells of atrioventricular node out of their refractory
period and is transmitted to ventricles; this is pattern of 2:1 block; note
that P-R interval following P_1 and P_3
is same

Fig. 8-4. Mechanism of 2:1 A-V block.

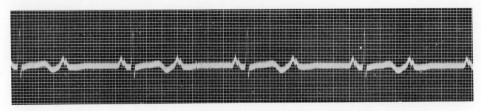

Fig. 8-5. 2:1 A-V block.

If one understands what happens in the A-V node in this type of block, the electrocardiographic pattern is easy to recognize.

1. A-V conducting tissues that are diseased become fatigued more quickly than normal.

2. Each passage of an impulse produces greater fatigue.

3. As a result, with each passage the exciting impulse is transmitted more and more slowly, so that the P-R interval becomes longer with each transmission.

4. Finally, the A-V tissues are so fatigued that they are not capable of transmitting an impulse at all. The sinus impulse arriving at this point finds the tissues completely refractory and the P wave is blocked.

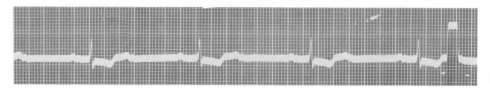

Fig. 8-6. 2:1 A-V block.

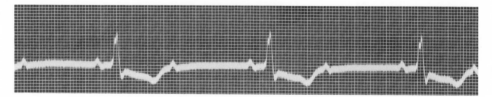

Fig. 8-7. 2:1 A-V block.

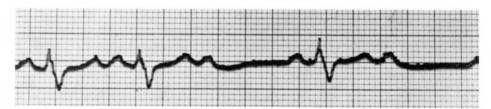

Fig. 8-8. Second-degree block, shifting from 3:2 to 2:1 ratio.

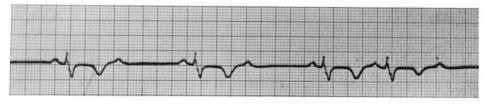

Fig. 8-9. Second-degree block, shifting from 2:1 to 3:2 ratio.

5. This period of nontransmission provides a rest for the A-V conducting tissues, and the next P wave following the blocked P will be conducted to the ventricles with the original short P-R interval.

The process just described is illustrated in Figs. 8-11 and 8-12. In Fig. 8-11 P_1 is conducted to the ventricles with a P-R interval of about .24 second. The next P-R

First sinus impulse passes through atrioventricular node; P-R interval may be normal or somewhat prolonged

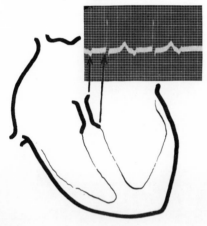

Fatigued by first transmission, cells of atrioventricular node take much longer to transmit second sinus impulse to ventricles

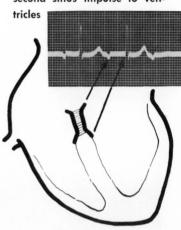

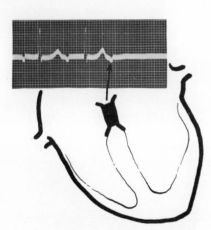

Further fatigued, cells of atrioventricular node completely incapable of transmitting third sinus impulse; it is therefore blocked

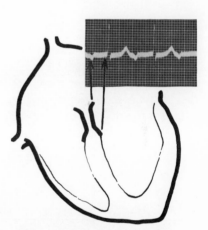

After rest period afforded by blocked beat, cells recover somewhat, and cycle starts over

Fig. 8-10. Wenckebach type of A-V block.

interval (P_2) is longer, about .36 second. The third P-R interval (P_3) is longer still, about .41 second. P_4 is superimposed on the T wave. This P wave is *not* followed by a ventricular complex; it is blocked in the A-V tissues. This completes the Wenckebach cycle, with gradual prolongation of the P-R interval until finally one P wave is blocked. Figs. 8-11 and 8-12 show the same cycle recurring a number of times.

Some variations of the Wenckebach phenomenon are important clinically.

Fig. 8-13 illustrates an important fact: the Wenckebach cycle may run through varying numbers of beats before one P wave is finally blocked. P_1, P_2, and P_3 are conducted before P_4 is blocked. P_5 and P_6 are then conducted, and P_7 is blocked. Thus, a four-beat cycle is followed by a three-beat cycle. This shift in ratio of conduction produces a grossly irregular pulse that could not be distinguished from atrial fibrillation by clinical examination.

Often a Wenckebach cycle starts with an A-V junctional escape beat. In the tracing shown in Fig. 8-14 P_1 comes just ahead of the ventricular complex. It is clear that this P wave could not possibly have reached the ventricles with this short a P-R interval, and the ventricular complex actually represents a junctional escape beat. The next P-R interval increases to .18 second, and the third P wave is blocked. Note, too, the rapid atrial rate (104) and the normal ventricular rate (about 80).

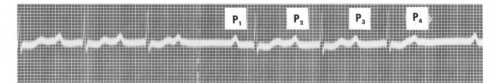

Fig. 8-11. Wenckebach type of A-V block.

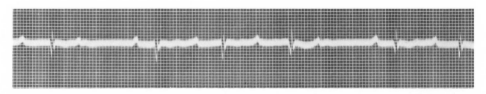

Fig. 8-12. Wenckebach type of A-V block.

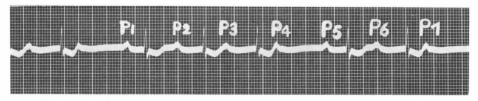

Fig. 8-13. Wenckebach type of A-V block. Note irregularity of the ventricular beat produced by change in length of cycles.

REMEMBER: *A-V block does not necessarily imply a slow ventricular rate. In many forms of A-V block the ventricular rate will be normal or rapid.*

This last point is illustrated in Fig. 8-15. Through most of this tracing the ventricular rate is about 106. The first Wenckebach cycle runs through six atrial beats and the second cycle runs through only two. The ventricular response, therefore, is rapid and grossly irregular, because of the drastic shift in degree of block.

In summary, the reasoning on which the diagnosis of Wenckebach A-V block is based is simple and logical:

1. Is the P-R interval changing? If it is, look for progressive prolongation of the P-R in successive beats.

2. If progressive prolongation of P-R in successive beats is present, look for a blocked P wave following the beat with the longest P-R interval.

3. The first P-R transmission following the blocked P wave should revert to a short P-R.

4. The ventricular rhythm will always be irregular for two reasons: first, there will be an occasional dropped ventricular response at the time of the blocked P wave, and, second, the changing P-R interval will produce a changing R-R interval. It seems contradictory, but as the P-R interval prolongs in Wenckebach A-V block, the R-R interval usually shortens. This is because the *rate of increase* of P-R interval almost always diminishes sharply after the second beat of the cycle. Thus a typical progression in P-R intervals in a Wenckebach cycle might run .16, .28, .32, .33. While the absolute length of the P-R increases with each beat, the amount of increase is less with each beat after the second beat of the cycle. Since the ventricular rate is based on the distance from R wave to R wave and not from R wave to P wave, the ventricular response is progressively more rapid until the blocked P wave produces a dropped ventricular beat. This characteristic shortening of R-R intervals in the presence of prolonging P-R intervals is sometimes a helpful sign in diagnosing Wenckebach type of A-V block. (Try working this out with a ruler, and the apparent paradox soon resolves itself.)

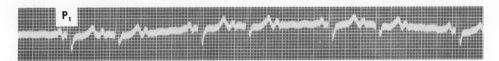

Fig. 8-14. Wenckebach type of A-V block. The ventricular beat following P_1 probably indicates a "nodal escape."

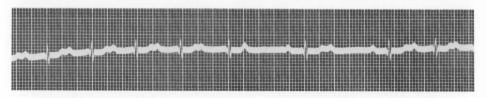

Fig. 8-15. Wenckebach type of A-V block. Note the rapid irregular ventricular rhythm.

This is the first arrhythmia presented with a changing P-R interval. As a rule of thumb, a changing P-R interval associated with a changing ventricular rhythm makes it likely that the mechanism is a Wenckebach A-V block. To confirm the diagnosis, go through the reasoning process listed above.

Mobitz Type 2 block*

Mobitz Type 2 block is easy to recognize but difficult to define. It is important because it usually implies a much more serious prognosis than the Wenckebach type of A-V block.

Mobitz described a type of block in which an occasional P wave was not conducted to the ventricles (Fig. 8-16). This blocking of an occasional P wave happens without any warning—that is, without any prolongation of P-R interval before the blocked P wave. The P-R interval of the conducted beats in the tracing may be normal or prolonged, *but it will be constant.* The P wave that is blocked is *not* premature; it is a sinus P wave at a normal interval that is not conducted to the ventricles. A precise definition of Mobitz Type 2 block would run something like this:

1. Two or more sinus impulses are conducted to the ventricles sequentially with the same P-R interval.
2. One sinus impulse is blocked, producing a P wave not followed by a ventricular complex.
3. After the blocked P wave, conduction from S-A node to ventricles resumes, with the same constant P-R interval as before the blocked P wave.

There is often confusion about 2:1 block as compared with Mobitz Type 2 block. The preceding definition makes it clear that 2:1 A-V block as defined earlier in this chapter is *not* true Mobitz Type 2 block, since in 2:1 block only one sinus impulse is conducted to the ventricles before the blocked P wave.

REMEMBER: *There must be two or more conducted sinus impulses with a constant P-R interval before the blocked P wave to constitute a true Mobitz Type 2 A-V block.*

---

*The words "Type 2" are appended to Mobitz's name when describing this type of block, since Mobitz also described the Wenckebach phenomenon, naming it "Type 1." It would probably be simpler if one used the word "Mobitz" to describe occasional blocking of P waves and "Wenckebach" to describe progressive prolongation of P-R interval, but common usage has produced the term "Mobitz Type 2" with which the student should be familiar.

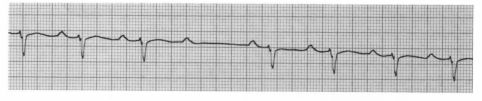

Fig. 8-16. Mobitz Type 2 block. Note the blocking of the third sinus P wave without any progressive prolongation of the P-R interval in the beats preceding the blocked P. This is characteristic of Mobitz Type 2 block. There is a prolonged P-R interval in the beats preceding the blocked P wave, *but the P-R interval is constant.* There is slight shortening of the P-R interval in the first sinus beat after the blocked P; all other beats before and after the blocked P wave manifest the same fixed P-R interval (.28 second). The slight shortening of the first P-R interval after the blocked P does not mean that a Wenckebach type of block is present. This is a common finding in true Mobitz Type 2 block.

This very precise definition is necessary, since recognition of Mobitz Type 2 block may be a life-and-death affair.

A 3:2 block, strictly speaking, falls within the class of Mobitz Type 2, since there are *two* conducted beats with a fixed P-R interval before the third P wave is blocked. Fig. 8-16 shows characteristic Mobitz Type 2 block with a prolonged but *fixed* P-R interval and with one nonconducted sinus P wave.

Mobitz Type 2 block very often implies block in the bundle branch system and, when seen in conjunction with a myocardial infarct, implies a much graver prognosis than the Wenckebach type of block.

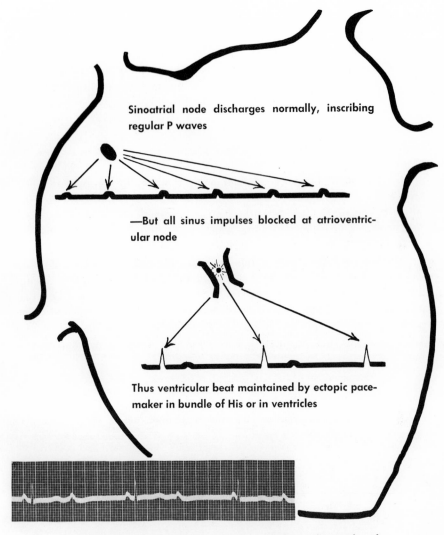

Sinoatrial node discharges normally, inscribing regular P waves

—But all sinus impulses blocked at atrioventricular node

Thus ventricular beat maintained by ectopic pacemaker in bundle of His or in ventricles

As a result, P waves and ventricular complexes disposed and superimposed at random with no consistent relationship to each other in EKG

Fig. 8-17. Complete A-V block.

Complete heart block

Complete heart block (Fig. 8-17) is the ultimate stage of disease of the A-V conducting system. The structures have completely ceased their function. No impulses pass from the atria to the ventricles, and life is maintained by an ectopic pacemaker in the bundle of His or in the ventricles that sets an independent rhythm for the ventricles. This independent rhythm is simply an idioventricular rhythm, and it is almost always slow and regular.

The atria and the ventricles each contract at their own independent rate. In the electrocardiogram P waves and ventricular complexes are inscribed in a completely irregular relationship. The P-R interval varies without any perceptible pattern, with P waves coming before, during, or after ventricular complexes, as chance will have it.

Fig. 8-18 illustrates the criteria for complete heart block.

1. The atrial and ventricular rates are *different:* the atrial rate is faster, the ventricular rate is slow and regular.

2. There is no consistent relation between P waves and ventricular complexes.

To decide whether block is partial or complete, inspect the tracing, noting the intervals between each P wave and the nearest succeeding ventricular complex. Ask yourself the following questions:

1. Is the P-R interval constant?

2. If it is not, does the P-R interval increase progressively, as in a Wenckebach phenomenon?

3. If it does not, does the relation of P waves to ventricular complexes vary widely, without any apparent pattern, with the P waves appearing irregularly before, during, and after the ventricular complexes?

4. Is the ventricular rhythm regular?

If these criteria are met, complete A-V block is present.

Another simple set of questions can be posed to distinguish Wenckebach A-V block and complete A-V block from other forms of A-V conduction failure.

1. Does the P-R interval change? If it does, the diagnosis will be either Wenckebach type of second-degree block or complete heart block, since for practical purposes these are the only two types of block in which the P-R interval changes.

2. If the answer to question 1 is "yes," ask whether the ventricular rhythm is

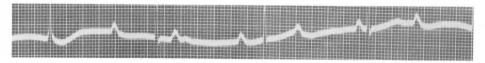

Fig. 8-18. Complete A-V block.

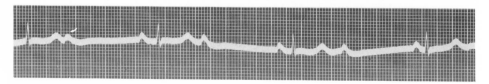

Fig. 8-19. Complete A-V block.

regular or not. In Wenckebach type of A-V block the ventricular rhythm is always *irregular,* because of the occasional blocked P waves and because of the changing P-R interval. In complete heart block, the ventricular rhythm is almost always regular, so that the combination of changing relation of P waves to ventricular complexes, with a regular ventricular rhythm, for practical purposes makes the diagnosis of complete A-V block.

Remember that with rare exceptions the ventricular rhythm is *regular* in complete A-V block. This is because of the inherently regular character of the A-V junctional or ventricular pacemakers that maintain the beat.

Figs. 8-19 to 8-21 illustrate complete heart block.

Atrioventricular block localized in the bundle branches

Disease or dysfunction of the A-V node can produce any of the types of block described so far. Disease or dysfunction of part or all of the ventricular bundle branch system may have precisely the same effect. This section will describe some criteria by which it is possible to detect A-V block in the bundle branch system with some accuracy.

In certain clinical situations it is very important to decide whether block is localized in the A-V node or in the bundle branch system.

1. A-V block within the bundle branch system is more likely to produce Stokes-Adams seizures than block within the A-V node.

2. The vagus nerve reaches and influences the A-V node, but it does not reach or influence the bundle branch system. Hence, A-V nodal block may result in part from vagal influence and may be ameliorated by antivagal drugs. Antivagal drugs will be ineffectual if the block is localized in the bundle branch system.

3. By noting the *progression of block* within the bundle branch system it is possible to select those patients who run the greatest risk of a Stokes-Adams seizure.

4. Block produced by digitalis will always be localized in the A-V node and not in the bundle branch system.

It is important to remember that tissue within the bundle branch system is susceptible to all the types of altered function found in the A-V node. Prolongation of conduction, intermittent conduction, or complete failure of conduction may be found

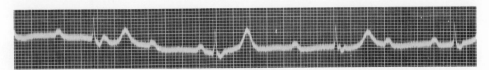

Fig. 8-20. Complete A-V block.

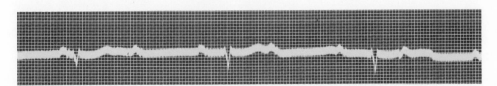

Fig. 8-21. Complete A-V block.

in the bundle branch system, resulting in first-, second-, or third-degree A-V block.

It is easy to grasp the patterns of block within the bundle branch system if one imagines a progression in severity.

1. Simple prolongation of conduction within bundle branch tissue may produce first-degree A-V block if the conduction delay is identical in both bundle branches. Picture an activating wave that has been normally propagated through the A-V node and bundle of His encountering *identical delay* in the left and right bundle branches, so that both ventricles are activated at the same time. Ventricular activation will still be normal, but the total distance from P wave to QRS complex will be prolonged. The result will be a prolonged P-R interval with a normal QRS complex—in other words, first-degree A-V block (Fig. 8-22). There is no way to differentiate this type of block from first-degree block in the A-V node except by bundle of His recording.

2. Complete block of one bundle branch means that A-V conduction can take place only through the other bundle branch. If transmission down the functioning bundle branch is slow, there will be prolongation of the P-R interval combined with a wide QRS complex, because of the complete block of the opposite bundle branch. Thus first-degree block with a bundle branch *block* may represent delayed conduction in the functioning bundle branch—first-degree block localized in the bundle branch system (Fig. 8-23).

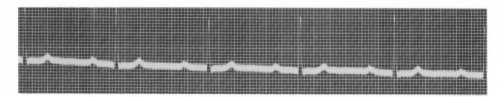

Fig. 8-22. First-degree A-V block with narrow QRS complex. The block here might be localized in the A-V node. It might also represent identical prolongation of conduction in both bundle branches, so that the activating wave reaching both ventricles followed a normal course but simply took a longer time than usual in transit down the two bundle branches. Differentiation between A-V block and first-degree delay in both bundle branches is not possible from this tracing alone.

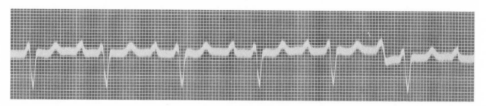

Fig. 8-23. First-degree A-V block with wide QRS complex (bundle branch block). Inspection of full electrocardiogram leads revealed that left bundle branch block was present. It is therefore possible that the prolonged P-R interval may be caused by delayed conduction through the right bundle branch, since this is now the only means by which an exciting wave can reach the ventricles from the atria. Delayed conduction down this one functioning bundle branch will therefore prolong the P-R interval. Prolonged P-R interval might also be caused by delayed conduction through the A-V node.

3. If one bundle branch is blocked and if transmission in the functioning bundle branch is delayed so that only every other atrial complex reaches the ventricles, the result will be 2:1 A-V block with a *wide ventricular complex* (Fig. 8-24).

4. Wenckebach delay in one bundle branch when the other bundle branch is completely blocked will produce a Wenckebach-type of P-R prolongation, again with a wide QRS complex (Fig. 8-25).

5. Mobitz Type 2 block is particularly likely to take place when one bundle branch is blocked and when the remaining bundle branch occasionally fails to conduct the P wave to the ventricles (Fig. 8-26).

6. Finally, complete block of both bundle branches will produce third-degree or complete A-V block—again, *with a wide QRS complex* (Fig. 8-27).

To summarize, the combination of bundle branch block with any type of A-V delay makes it possible that the source of the A-V block is in the bundle branch system.

Fascicular block within the bundle branch system

In recent years it has been established that the left bundle divides into two separate functional units or fascicles early in its course through the ventricle. One

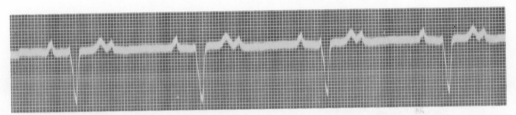

Fig. 8-24. 2:1 A-V block with bundle branch block. Lead V$_1$ reveals that left bundle branch block is present. Conduction from atria to ventricles can take place only down the right bundle branch. The 2:1 A-V block may therefore represent failure of the right bundle branch to conduct every alternate P wave, because of a prolonged refractory period in the bundle branch tissues. On the other hand, the block may be localized in the A-V node. The combination of second-degree A-V block with block of one bundle branch raises the possibility that the A-V delay is caused by intermittent failure of conduction in the other bundle branch.

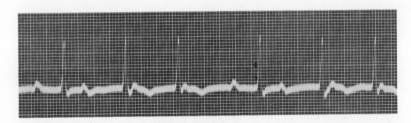

Fig. 8-25. Wenckebach type of A-V block in the presence of bundle branch block. Note the wide S wave that produces a QRS .12 second in width. Right bundle branch block is present. A typical Wenckebach type of progressive P-R prolongation culminating in a blocked P wave is apparent. The Wenckebach phenomenon is much more common in the A-V node than in the bundle branch system, but it can occur in the bundle branches. Since the left bundle branch is the only communication between atria and ventricles here, it is possible that the progressive P-R prolongation represents progressive fatigue of the left bundle branch, a form of bifascicular block. On the other hand, the block may be localized in the A-V node, which is statistically more likely.

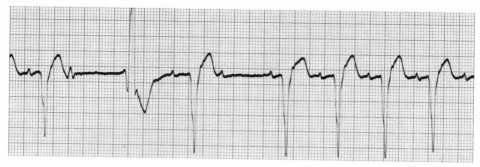

Fig. 8-26. Mobitz Type 2 block with bundle branch block. This is a complex arrhythmia that includes an episode of Mobitz Type 2 block. Note the wide QRS complexes in lead V_1. Left bundle branch block is present. Second visible P wave is a premature P wave that is not conducted to the ventricles. In the pause following this a ventricular ectopic beat escapes. The first P-R interval following the ventricular ectopic beat is slightly prolonged, probably because the A-V node is fatigued by retrograde conduction from the ventricular ectopic beat. (This is an example of "concealed conduction.") The next sinus P wave is not conducted to the ventricles. Subsequently, a normal sinus rhythm resumes. The combination of Mobitz Type 2 block with bundle branch block makes it very likely that the site of A-V block is in the two bundle branches; that is, with the left bundle branch already known to be blocked, the right bundle branch simply failed to conduct one P wave to the ventricles.

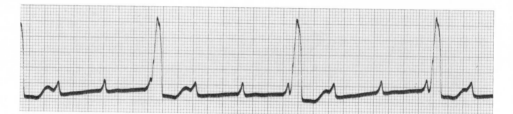

Fig. 8-27. Complete A-V block with a slow ventricular pacemaker. It is very likely that the block in this case lies below the A-V node in the upper portions of both bundle branches.

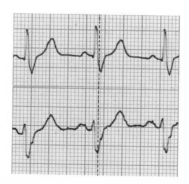

Fig. 8-28. Method of measuring frontal plane axis in the presence of right bundle branch block. Since the first .07 second of the QRS represents activation of the left ventricle, this point is taken to measure axis before beginning of inscription of the slow "blocked" wave traversing the right ventricle. The dotted line here indicates about the point at which the axis measurement should be determined in the presence of right bundle branch block.

fascicle conducts anteriorly or superiorly while the other conducts posteriorly or inferiorly. Either of these fascicles may be blocked for any of the usual reasons; as a result, isolated activation of the left ventricle will take place along the opposite, functioning fascicle.

Fortunately for diagnostic purposes, it is easy to tell when one fascicle of the left bundle branch is blocked. Electrically speaking, the fascicles point in "opposite directions." It is necessary only to know how to calculate axis direction in the frontal plane to distinguish block of one of the two fascicles of the left bundle branch.

Isolated conduction along the posterior fascicle (anterior fascicular block) produces extreme left axis deviation (−45 degrees or greater).

Isolated conduction along the anterior fascicle (posterior fascicular block) produces extreme right axis deviation (+120 degrees or greater).

Anterior fascicular block is therefore diagnosed when the fontal plane axis is −45 degrees or leftward, the QRS is slightly widened (.11 second), and the frontal plane leads show a qR configuration in lead I and an rS in lead III (counterclockwise rotation in the frontal planes). The QRS is slightly wider than normal because of the slow retrograde activation of the blocked fascicular area of the left ventricle.

While anterior fascicular block is an absolute and positive diagnosis when these criteria are met, *posterior* fascicular block is a diagnosis of exclusion; it can be diagnosed only when other causes of extreme right axis deviation have been ruled out (pulmonic stenosis, pulmonary hypertension, mitral stenosis, congenital lesions with left-to-right shunt, and the like).

Posterior fascicular block is therefore diagnosed when extreme right axis deviation is combined with a slightly wide QRS (.11) and a frontal lead configuration with an rS in lead I and a qR in lead III (clockwise rotation in the frontal leads). Remember that other causes of extreme right axis deviation must be ruled out before the diagnosis of posterior fascicular block is made.

The sudden appearance of extreme left or extreme right axis in the frontal plane may imply that one of the fascicles of the left bundle branch has been blocked. This type of conduction abnormality is often termed "hemiblock" or fascicular block. There will be no change in the P-R interval.

Bifascicular block

The combination of complete right bundle branch block with block of either of the fascicles of the left bundle branch is called bifascicular block. The diagnosis is simple: it is based on detection of extreme left or extreme right axis deviation in the presence of right bundle branch block.

NOTE: *When right bundle branch block is present, activation of the left ventricle is recorded in the initial part of the QRS complex, while the slow activation of the right ventricle is recorded in the terminal portion.* Since it is the direction of left ventricular activation that tells which fascicle is blocked, the initial (.07 second) part of the QRS must be used to derive the axis (Fig. 8-28). Figs. 8-29 and 8-30 give examples of anterior and posterior fascicular block in the presence of right bundle branch block.

Trifascicular block

When there is any delay in A-V transmission in the presence of bifascicular block, the assumption is that the A-V delay lies in the remaining functioning fascicle. The term "trifascicular block" is therefore used when first- or second-degree block of any type appears in the presence of bifascicular block.

When bifascicular block is followed by complete heart block, the assumption is that bilateral bundle branch block is the anatomic diagnosis and that in fact complete trifascicular block is present.

Summary

A-V block of any degree may be localized in the A-V node or in the bundle branch system.

First- or second-degree A-V block with narrow QRS complexes may be localized in the A-V node or in the bundle of His. First- or second-degree block with wide QRS complexes may be localized in the bundle branch system. Mobitz Type 2 block with wide QRS complexes is usually localized in the bundle branch system.

Complete A-V block is localized in the bundle branch system from 30% to 70%

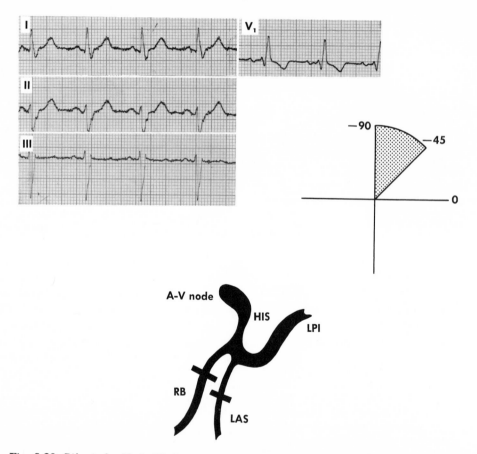

Fig. 8-29. Bifascicular block. Block of the anterior fascicle of the left bundle branch, together with block of the right bundle. Note the characteristic right bundle branch appearance in lead V₁. Measuring the frontal plane axis at the .07 second point of the QRS in leads I, II, and III indicates extreme left axis. When the anterior fascicle of the left bundle is blocked, isolated conduction through the left posterior-inferior fascicle will give an extreme left axis somewhere between −45 and −90 degrees.

of the time, based on various studies of the bundle of His. When the QRS complex is wide, the block is very likely to be localized in the bundle branch system. *A narrow QRS complex means that the ventricular pacemaker is in the A-V nodal junction or in the bundle of His;* the block must therefore lie above that point.

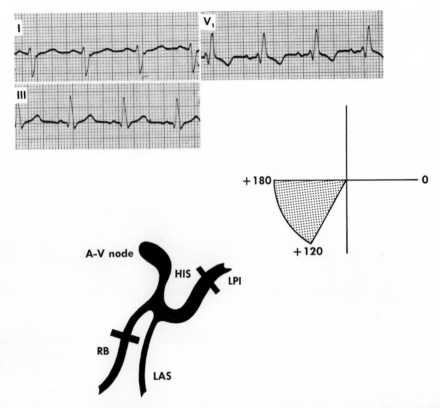

Fig. 8-30. Posterior fascicular block in the presence of right bundle branch block. Lead V_1 shows the characteristic deformity of right bundle branch block. Leads I and III reveal extreme right axis in the frontal plane. When the left posterior fascicle of the left bundle is blocked, isolated conduction through the left anterior-superior fascicle will produce extreme right axis somewhere between +120 and +180 degrees. Again, remember to measure the axis at the .07 second point of the QRS.

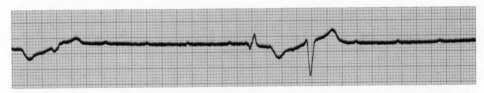

Fig. 8-31. Stokes-Adams episode. A high degree of A-V block is present, with failure of ventricular systole for periods of several seconds. This disorder of rhythm appeared abruptly in a patient who had had 2:1 A-V block with wide QRS complexes. During these periods of asystole, extreme vertigo and sometimes syncope were noted. Stokes-Adams episodes—meaning periods of asystole caused by a high degree of A-V block—are very dangerous and are often fatal.

The appearance of any type of A-V delay in the presence of bifascicular block implies that the delay is the result of faulty conduction through the remaining viable fascicle of the bundle branch system—in other words, trifascicular block.

Remember that complete A-V block with wide QRS complexes may also be the result of block in the A-V node with complete block of one bundle branch.

SYMPTOMS

The only symptoms directly related to A-V block are syncope or vertigo associated with complete cessation of ventricular systole for a period of several seconds, that is, Stokes-Adams seizures (Fig. 8-31). Sometimes these will be obvious, with complete loss of consciousness, but often short periods of asystole will be described as "severe dizziness," "swimming in the head," "going blind for a few seconds," and so on, through many variations of the basic theme of inadequate cerebral blood flow.

When symptoms suggestive of Stokes-Adams seizures accompany electrocardiographic evidence of A-V block, the most careful investigation is warranted. These simple rules may prove helpful:

1. When Stokes-Adams episodes accompany complete A-V block, the assumption is that the conduction delay is the cause of syncope, and a permanent pacemaker is implanted. *Rule out the other causes of syncope.* Be sure, for example, that ischemic cerebral disease or postural hypotension are not the real causes of the symptom.

2. When the Stokes-Adams attack accompanies second-degree A-V block, *study the patient to see whether an increase in heart rate increases the severity of the block, with production of significant periods of ventricular asystole.* This can be done in three ways:

a. Have the patient exercise on a treadmill or other device while his electrocardiogram is monitored continuously. This is the simplest and often the best mode of diagnosis.

b. If the patient cannot exercise, introduce a pacing catheter into the right atrium and drive the heart at gradually increasing rates, observing the electrocardiogram continuously.

c. Have the patient wear a continuously recording 12-hour electrocardiogram monitor (the Holter monitor), which permits playback of the electrocardiogram on a scanning device to detect periods of asystole.

Recording of bundle of His potentials has been tremendously informative on a research basis, but it is rare that this type of recording gives pragmatically useful information. What the physician needs to know can be summed up in two questions, both of which can almost always be answered by the diagnostic procedures outlined:

1. Does the degree of block increase spontaneously to a dangerous level, with periods of asystole that may threaten life?

2. Does increase in rate increase the degree of block to a dangerous level?

It is possible that block below the bundle of His—that is, in the H-P interval—might be concealed because of a short A-H interval, so that on adding the sinus-His and His-ventricular intervals, the total P-R in the conventional electrocardiogram would be normal. This has been documented, but it is very rare. Such a case would represent a genuine indication for bundle of His recording.

Remember that Stokes-Adams seizures are very often fatal. A patient who has had one attack should be subjected to thorough study. A patient who has had more than one attack is in great danger of sudden death and should be treated accordingly.

CLINICAL DIAGNOSIS

Complete A-V block is the *only* arrhythmia in which a correct diagnosis can be established at the bedside. Three features of the physical examination make this possible:

1. The independent atrial rhythm will produce "a" waves in the jugular venous pulse, which will almost always be more rapid than the ventricular rate. There will be no consistent relation between the jugular "a" waves and the ventricular beat as measured by palpation or auscultation.

2. Occasionally, the atria will contract against a closed tricuspid valve. This will produce a large "a" wave in the jugular vein, often called a "cannon 'a' wave."

3. The first heart sound will vary in intensity from beat to beat, ranging from faint to very loud, with a booming or snapping quality. The reason for this variation lies in the different degree of opening of the mitral and tricuspid valves and the time of ventricular systole. Since there is no relation between atrial and ventricular systole in complete A-V block, the A-V valves may be in any position from closed to widely open at the time of ventricular systole. If a P wave happens to come at just the right distance before the QRS complex, the mitral and tricuspid valves will open to exactly the right degree to make a maximal sound when closing, thus producing the intermittent, peculiarly loud, first heart and sound characteristic of complete A-V block.

Vagal fibers reach and influence the A-V node. They do *not* reach or influence the ventricular conducting tissues. As a result, an ectopic pacemaker in the ventricles will *not* be influenced by atropine and will be influenced very little by changes in posture or by exertion. Characteristically, an ectopic pacemaker in the ventricular tissues will be slow, regular, and stable. On the other hand, an ectopic pacemaker in the A-V node *will* be influenced by vagal effect and hence will show a speeding of rate with atropine, exercise, change in position, and the like. Pacemakers in the A-V junctional tissue are characteristically more rapid than those in the ventricles. These rather simple clinical observations may often help make the distinction between complete A-V block in the bundle branch system and A-V block in the A-V node with block of one bundle branch, which produces a wide QRS.

TREATMENT
First-degree block

First-degree A-V block, per se, is not a threat to life and does not require specific treatment. Diagnosis of first-degree A-V block may help the clinician confirm the presence of acute carditis of some type, detect the onset of drug toxicity (digitalis, quinidine, and so on), detect electrolyte abnormality such as an elevated serum potassium, or, at times, detect pathology caused by coronary artery disease or other degenerative processes.

Second-degree block

Second-degree A-V block is significant and requires treatment in a few specific situations:

1. In the presence of an acute myocardial infarct
2. When the ventricular rate is so slow that cardiac output is significantly compromised
3. When second-degree A-V block is associated with Stokes-Adams attacks

Complete block

Complete A-V block requires treatment in three specific clinical situations:

1. When complete A-V block appears acutely following a myocardial infarct
2. When Stokes-Adams episodes are diagnosed or suspected
3. When the ventricular rate is so slow that cardiac output is compromised

When block is localized in the A-V node, drug therapy may be useful. When block is localized in the bundle branch system, drug therapy directed specifically at the block is probably useless.

Certain simple, logical rules govern indications for treatment in A-V block.

1. Any patient with second- or third-degree A-V block with what seem to be Stokes-Adams episodes should have a permanent pacemaker implanted. (See Chapter 20.) Stokes-Adams episodes are frequently fatal, and there is no justification for withholding definitive treatment.

2. Patients with second-degree A-V block with significant slowing of ventricular rate who have minimal symptoms that may be related to the block may reasonably be given a trial of medical therapy. It is well to evaluate the effect of atropine acutely, administering 0.5 mg intravenously every 4 to 6 hours for three doses. If vagal effect is important in genesis of the block, this acute atropinization will diminish the degree of block and may abolish A-V block entirely. Atropine is not suitable for prolonged use because of the side effects attending full atropinization.

Isoproterenol, sublingually, may be tried in this same group of patients. From 5 to 15 mg may be given sublingually three or four times a day, or more often if symptoms warrant and tolerance permits. Chronic use of isoproterenol may produce significant symptomatic benefit in a small, select group of patients.

When second- or third-degree block appears acutely in a patient who has suffered a myocardial infarct, a temporary transvenous pacemaker should be introduced into the right ventricle without delay. (See Chapter 20.)

In a patient with impaired cardiac function with permanent second-degree A-V block and significant slowing of ventricular rate, a trial of transvenous pacing should be carried on to see how much the patient's hemodynamic state is improved. If cardiac output and oxygen uptake can be made to increase significantly during a temporary period of pacing, permanent implantation of a pacemaker is indicated. This kind of testing can be done only in a laboratory equipped to measure cardiac output and oxygen uptake and should not be attempted in any unit not prepared to carry out both measurements.

Complete heart block associated with Stokes-Adams episodes or even with symptoms suggesting Stokes-Adams episodes is an absolute indication for implantation of a permanent pacemaker.

Complete A-V block without significant symptoms is a "gray area." It is still not clear whether the morbidity and mortality of pacemaker implantation outweigh the risk of a fatal first Stokes-Adams episode, which is statistically very small.

Patients with compromised cardiac function and a slow ventricular rate associated with complete heart block should have a permanent pacemaker implanted whether Stokes-Adams episodes have been present or not, since the patient will certainly require the increase in cardiac output that can be accomplished by pacing at an optimal rate. In some patients with severe cardiac damage who require every possible augmentation of output, it may still be advisable to consider atrial synchronized pacing—the type of pacemaker that synchronizes the atrial and ventricular beats and produces the maximum cardiac output per beat.

REFERENCES

Brown, R., Hunt, D., and Sloman, J.: The natural history of atrioventricular conduction defects in acute myocardial infarction, Am. Heart J. **78**:460-466, 1969.

Corne, R., and Mathewson, F.: Congenital complete atrioventricular heart block: a 25 year follow-up study, Am. J. Cardiol. **29**:413-415, 1972.

Dreifus, L. S., and Watanabe, Y.: Localization and significance of atrioventricular block, Am. Heart J. **82**:435-438, 1971.

Hackel, D., and Estes, E., Jr.: Pathologic features of atrioventricular and intraventricular conduction disturbances in acute myocardial infarction, Circulation **43**:977-979, 1971.

Hatle, L., and Rokseth, R.: Conservative treatment of AV block in acute myocardial infarction, Brit. Heart J. **33**:595-600, 1971.

Langendorf, R., Cohen, H., and Gozo, E., Jr.: Observations on second degree atrioventricular block, including new criteria for the differential diagnosis between Type I and Type II block, Am. J. Cardiol. **29**:111-119, 1972.

Pryor, R., and Blount, S. G., Jr.: The clinical significance of true left axis deviation: left intraventricular blocks, Am. Heart J. **72**:391-413, 1966.

Rosen, K., and others: Mobitz Type II block without bundle-branch block, Circulation **44**:1111-1119, 1971.

Rosen, K., and others: Electrophysiological significance of first degree atrioventricular block with intraventricular conduction disturbance, Circulation **43**:491-502, 1971.

Rosenbaum, M.: The hemiblocks: diagnostic criteria and clinical significance, Mod. Concept. Cardiovasc. Dis. **39**:141-146, 1970.

Rosenbaum, M. B., and others: Intraventricular trifascicular blocks: review of the literature and classification, Am. Heart J. **78**:306-317, 1969.

9 Atrial fibrillation

Atrial fibrillation is the most common of the major arrhythmias. No one can practice medicine long without encountering the grossly irregular pulse of atrial fibrillation.

MECHANISM

Imagine yourself throwing handfuls of pebbles into a pond as rapidly as possible. The surface of the water would be crisscrossed by hundreds of ripples, irregular in shape, size, and distribution, intersecting, cancelling, and reinforcing with no fixed pattern.

This is a good picture of atrial fibrillation. The chambers are traversed by hundreds of fine, rapid wave fronts. The atrial muscle does not contract—it simply quivers.

The A-V node is bombarded by hundreds of these tiny impulses every minute. Most of them will find the node in its refractory state and will go no farther. Now and then a wave will happen to strike the node when it is ready to conduct (that is, when it is out of its refractory state) and the ventricles will then be stimulated (Fig. 9-1).

This hit-or-miss stimulation produces the characteristic, completely irregular ventricular rhythm.

Fig. 9-2 illustrates the mechanism of atrial fibrillation. The tiny waves, labeled *f*, are produced by the fibrillating atria. The irregular spacing of the ventricular complexes is obvious.

CAUSES

Any disease capable of producing ischemia or hypertrophy of the atria can produce atrial fibrillation. In younger persons (under 50 years of age) the common causes of atrial fibrillation are congenital heart disease and rheumatic heart disease with mitral involvement. Mitral stenosis in particular gives rise to this arrhythmia because of the drastic rise in left atrial pressure and massive left atrial hypertrophy that attend this valve defect.

In persons over 50 years of age disease of the coronary arteries is very often the cause. Ischemia of the atrial syncytium is the inciting factor in these patients.

In patients of any age, thyrotoxicosis may cause atrial fibrillation. Whenever this arrhythmia is detected in the absence of signs of organic heart disease the physician must check carefully for an overactive thyroid. The cardiac manifestations of hyperthyroidism may precede other clinical signs by months or years.

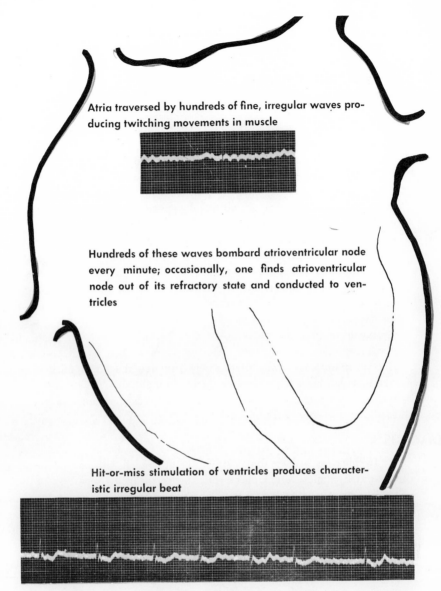

Atria traversed by hundreds of fine, irregular waves producing twitching movements in muscle

Hundreds of these waves bombard atrioventricular node every minute; occasionally, one finds atrioventricular node out of its refractory state and conducted to ventricles

Hit-or-miss stimulation of ventricles produces characteristic irregular beat

Fig. 9-1. Atrial fibrillation.

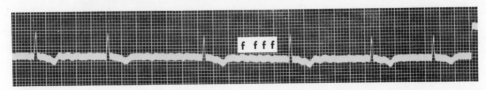

f f f

Fig. 9-2. Atrial fibrillation. The fibrillary impulses traversing the atria are represented by the fine irregular waves labeled *f.*

SIGNIFICANCE

Atrial fibrillation is not a benign arrhythmia! The reasons are simple:

1. Cardiac output always falls in the presence of atrial fibrillation as compared to the output in the presence of sinus rhythm in the same patient at the same time. Remember that "atrial kick" produces a "supercharging" effect on the ventricles, with the net result of increasing the amount of blood pumped per stroke of the heart. A healthy individual has mechanisms to compensate for this lack, but in a patient with significant heart disease the absence of a synchronized atrial beat may produce a critical drop in cardiac output. It is common to see a fall of as much as 25% in the cardiac output when atrial fibrillation interrupts a normal sinus rhythm.

2. Excessively rapid bombardment of the A-V node by the fibrillating atria will result in a very rapid, irregular ventricular rate and rhythm. Ventricular pumping action becomes inefficient and congestive failure will inevitably follow.

3. A very large percentage of patients with chronic atrial fibrillation will develop mural thrombi in the atria and atrial appendages. These mural thrombi will subsequently discharge emboli that may cripple or kill. It has been noted that the greatest danger of systemic embolization occurs during the first 6 months of atrial fibrillation, but some danger persists as long as atrial fibrillation is present, particularly in a patient with an enlarged atrium. (It has been noted that about one out of three patients with atrial enlargement and chronic atrial fibrillation will ultimately suffer arterial emboli that may be lethal. Thus atrial fibrillation in this context is a more dangerous disease than untreated syphilis.*)

Whenever possible, therefore, the arrhythmia should be terminated and a sinus rhythm should be maintained. There are times when it will predictably *not* be possible to maintain a sinus rhythm, even though the atrial fibrillation is temporarily terminated, and in these patients therapy should simply be directed at maintaining a normal ventricular rate consistent with optimal cardiac function. (Note indications for cardioversion later in this chapter.)

DIAGNOSIS

In this case, bedside diagnosis can be attempted with more hope of success than in other arrhythmias. Again, check with an electrocardiogram!

The grossly irregular ventricular pulse is usually obvious to every senior medical student. At very rapid rates this may be difficult to detect. In other instances, complete block in the A-V node will produce a regular ventricular rhythm while the atria are fibrillating.

Presence of a *pulse deficit is helpful*. This means that the physician hears more beats at the apex than can be counted at the radial pulse at the same time. Some beats come so early in diastole that very little blood is ejected from the ventricles, not enough to produce a palpable pulse, hence the difference.

This same phenomenon may be detected in another way. When the blood pressure is taken, some beats will register with a higher pressure than others. Those coming later in diastole, with complete ventricular filling, will produce a higher systolic pressure than will those coming earlier. As the pressure is dropped in the cuff, a few beats

---

*In the preantibiotic era, only about one out of four cases of untreated syphilis ever progressed to the point at which the patient had significant cardiovascular or central nervous system syphilis, hence the startling but accurate comparison.

may be heard; for example, at a systolic level of 150, more can be heard at a level of 130, and all beats can be heard at a level of 110.

Every grossly irregular pulse is not atrial fibrillation. To treat some of the other arrhythmias as you would treat atrial fibrillation might be fatal. Take an electrocardiogram!

Electrocardiographic diagnosis

If you remember the mechanism, the electrocardiographic pattern is simple.

1. The S-A node is not discharging—*no P waves are seen.*
2. The atrial muscle is fibrillating—*fine fibrillary waves are seen in one or more leads.*
3. Conduction to the ventricles is haphazard—*the ventricular complexes appear at grossly irregular intervals.*

Fig. 9-3 illustrates atrial fibrillation with all of the characteristics just mentioned.

When the ventricular rate is very rapid, the rhythm may seem nearly regular. Careful inspection of the tracing shown in Fig. 9-4 will disclose the irregular spacing of the ventricular complexes. No P waves are seen. The rate is so rapid and the amplitude of the fibrillary waves is so low that these are not seen.

Conduction through the A-V node may be slow. Drugs such as digitalis and quinidine may produce this effect; so can organic disease of the A-V node. A slow rate does not rule out fibrillation (Fig. 9-5).

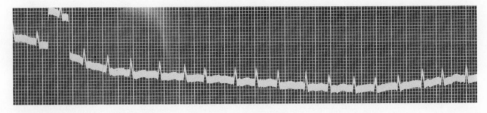

Fig. 9-3. Atrial fibrillation.

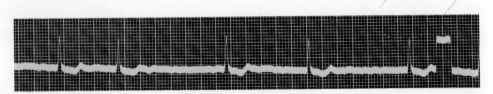

Fig. 9-4. Atrial fibrillation with rapid ventricular rate.

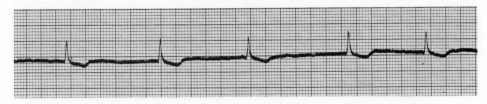

Fig. 9-5. Atrial fibrillation with slow ventricular rate (following digitalization).

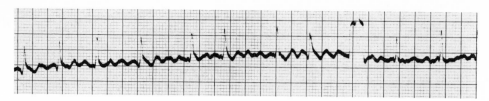

Fig. 9-6. Coarse atrial fibrillation.

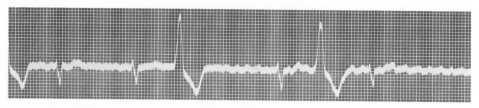

Fig. 9-7. Atrial fibrillation interrupted by premature ventricular beats.

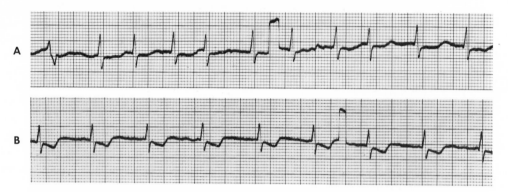

Fig. 9-8. A, Atrial fibrillation. **B,** Same patient after digitalization. Complete block is present in the A-V node: the atria are still fibrillating but the ventricular rhythm is now maintained by a pacemaker in the A-V junction or in the common bundle of His above its bifurcation.

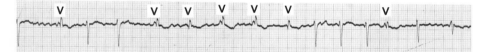

Fig. 9-9. Idioventricular rhythm appearing during atrial fibrillation. The wide beats labeled *V* represent the escape of a ventricular ectopic pacemaker during a period when the conduction of fibrillary waves from atria to ventricles had slowed, probably because of digitalis effect in the A-V node. There is therefore a period of complete A-V block with an idioventricular rhythm, even though it is brief, lasting only a few seconds. Note other isolated ventricular ectopic beats from the same focus.

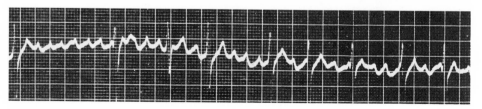

Fig. 9-10. Flutter-fibrillation.

Fibrillary waves may be very "coarse," that is, they may be large, relatively slow, and almost regular for short periods, as shown in Fig. 9-6. The irregularity of spacing of the fibrillary waves is obvious if one measures for several seconds.

Atrial fibrillation may be interrupted by ventricular premature beats (Fig. 9-7).

Complete block in the A-V node may stop all transmissions from atria to ventricles. The tracing shown in Fig. 9-8, *A*, is typical of atrial fibrillation. The tracing shown in Fig. 9-8, *B*, taken a few days later, shows that complete block in the A-V node has developed. The ventricular rhythm has become regular. Since no impulses from the fibrillating atria can now reach the ventricles, the rhythm is maintained by a pacemaker in the A-V node, the bundle of His, or the ventricles. In this case, the configuration of the ventricular complexes shows that the pacemaker lies above the bifurcation of the bundle of His, possibly in the A-V junction (because of the normal configuration of the ventricular complexes). Such a rhythm is often called an "idioventricular" rhythm even though the pacemaker may actually lie in the A-V junction. It is characteristically *regular*.

Fig. 9-9 illustrates a brief idioventricular rhythm interrupting atrial fibrillation. The beats labeled *V* all arise in an ectopic focus in the ventricles and for almost 4 seconds (in the center of the tracing) a true idioventricular rhythm is present. This kind of regular escape rhythm interrupting atrial fibrillation is practically always the result of digitalis intoxication.

There are two therapeutic and diagnostic morals to be drawn from Figs. 9-8 and 9-9. Fig. 9-8 illustrates the fact that restoration of a regular rhythm in the presence of atrial fibrillation does not always mean that normal sinus rhythm has been restored. An inefficient ectopic junctional rhythm may actually be present. Fig. 9-9 underscores the idea that complete block in the A-V node may appear for short periods during atrial fibrillation and would be extremely difficult to detect without an electrocardiogram by any but the most skilled cardiologist.

Atrial fibrillation may occur in short paroxysms, interrupting a sinus mechanism. Fibrillation may persist for seconds, days, or a lifetime.

FLUTTER-FIBRILLATION

Sometimes fibrillary waves are very large and nearly regular. They can be measured with the calipers for short periods and will be found to be uniform. After a few seconds this regularity disappears and the timing and contour of the waves change, making it clear that this cannot be a true flutter (Fig. 9-10).

This can be called coarse fibrillation or flutter-fibrillation. It is treated in the same manner as any fibrillation.

TREATMENT

Treatment has one of two goals:
1. Conversion of the atrial fibrillation to a sinus mechanism
2. Slowing of the ventricular rate to produce optimal cardiac function

Conversion to sinus rhythm

Atrial fibrillation can be converted to sinus rhythm by administration of quinidine or by electroversion. When quinidine was the only means of conversion, there was much disagreement about proper indications for this procedure. Since the introduction of electroversion a vast body of data has accumulated, and it is now possible to make specific statements about the indications for cardioversion and the dangers of the procedure.

As Doctor Lown, the originator of electroversion, has pointed out, the best way to describe the indications for cardioversion is to state when the procedure should *not* be carried out. Two sentences of simple, colloquial English can serve as maxims:

1. Do not convert a patient from atrial fibrillation to sinus rhythm unless the patient has a reasonable chance of staying converted.
2. Do not convert patients when the risk of cardioversion is greater than the benefit.

Patients who may reasonably be expected to maintain a normal sinus rhythm once converted fall into a few subcategories.

1. Patients with valvular heart disease accompanied by atrial fibrillation may be reasonably expected to maintain a normal sinus rhythm *after* the valve lesion has been repaired and the cause of the fibrillation thus removed. Cardioversion should therefore be attempted about 2 months after corrective valve surgery.

2. Thyrotoxic patients with atrial fibrillation who have been rendered euthyroid by medical management may reasonably be expected to maintain a normal sinus rhythm once converted. Therefore, if a thyrotoxic patient has reached euthyroid levels and if atrial fibrillation persists, cardioversion should be attempted.

3. Hypertensive heart disease and alcoholic myocardiopathy are two types of heart disease in which the cause of the disease and of the arrhythmia can be removed or abated. Therefore, if atrial fibrillation persists after a period of adequate control of blood pressure or of abstinence from alcohol, cardioversion may reasonably be attempted.

4. "Lone" atrial fibrillation—atrial fibrillation in a patient without other evidence of heart disease—is considered a benign entity by some writers and is not thought to constitute an indication for cardioversion. I feel that lone atrial fibrillation is benign only in individuals pursuing sedentary lives. Patients working at the moderate to strenuous levels of activity will almost certainly feel some effects of atrial fibrillation and will perform better and will feel better if a sinus rhythm is restored. Cardioversion may therefore be reasonably attempted in this group.

5. In rare patients with atrial fibrillation caused by uncorrectable heart disease it may be possible to maintain a normal sinus rhythm, with consequent improved cardiac output, for 6 or 8 months following each cardioversion. *If* maintenance of maximal output is critical and if the sinus rhythm can be maintained for a significant period (6 months or longer), cardioversion may properly be attempted.

Excessive risk with cardioversion

Excessive risk with cardioversion is found in the following:

1. Patients with any significant degree of A-V block
2. Elderly patients (70 to 75 years of age or older)
3. Patients with a previous history of a sick sinus. (See Chapter 14.) These are patients who may have had paroxysms of rapid ectopic atrial rhythm alternating with periods of very slow sinus rhythm, or sinus bradycardia. If such a patient begins fibrillating, termination of the arrhythmia by cardioversion carries a high risk.
4. Patients with chronic atrial fibrillation of several years' standing who have cardiac enlargement or uncorrectable heart disease
5. Patients who cannot take quinidine to maintain a normal sinus rhythm once it is established

Procedure

With these indications and dangers firmly in mind and with the patient properly selected, electroversion may be attempted. Some simple rules govern the procedure.

If the patient has suffered a previous embolus from the fibrillating atria or if the patient has an enlarged atrium that makes embolism more likely, anticoagulants should be used before cardioversion. It is interesting that embolism following cardioversion does *not* take place at the time of conversion to sinus rhythm: discharge of an embolus from the atrium takes place when and if the newly restored sinus rhythm ends and atrial fibrillation resumes. In these patients I begin carefully controlled anticoagulant therapy 1 month prior to the attempt at cardioversion. I continue anticoagulants for 2 weeks after cardioversion.

The day before cardioversion the patient is given 200 mg of quinidine at 2-hour intervals for eight doses. In some patients normal sinus rhythm will resume simply as a result of the quinidine and no further measures are necessary. The patient is anesthetized with intravenous diazepam and electroversion is attempted. (See Chapter 21.)

Quinidine cardioversion

If for some reason the physician does not wish to use electroversion, quinidine may be employed. I prefer relatively small doses of quinidine given at relatively frequent intervals—100 mg hourly or 200 mg every 2 hours over a period of 12 hours—with careful monitoring of pulse, blood pressure, and electrocardiogram throughout. A total dose of 2 to 3 gm may be given in 24 hours, always with very careful observation and, if possible, with measurement of blood levels after 12 hours of therapy. A blood level of 10 mg/liter of quinidine is almost certain to be toxic and is an indication for discontinuance of therapy until safer levels, in the range of 4 to 8 mg/liter, are reached.

The watchwords for the physician using quinidine to terminate any arrhythmia are "careful observation" and "caution." I feel that the deaths associated with quinidine administration have very often resulted from excessive doses and inadequate observation for signs of toxicity.

Maintenance of sinus rhythm

Once a normal sinus rhythm has been restored, it is customary to attempt to maintain the rhythm with oral quinidine. Two hundred milligrams three or four times a day will usually suffice.

Slowing of ventricular rate to ensure optimal cardiac performance

Digitalis slows the ventricular rate in atrial fibrillation by inducing partial block in the A-V node. Digitalis is used specifically to produce a slower, more efficient ventricular beat. *Digitalis does not, per se, change the fibrillary process.* In fact, the atria will fibrillate more rapidly after digitalization than before.

Sometimes a patient who has been fibrillating will convert to a sinus mechanism after digitalization. This is a secondary effect caused by the fact that digitalis increases the efficiency of the ventricular beat, thereby improving coronary perfusion and presumably improving oxygenation of the atrial tissues, as well as dropping left atrial pressure.

When conversion cannot be achieved, digitalis is excellent for prolonged management and, with its aid, a patient suffering from chronic atrial fibrillation may carry on a reasonably normal existence for many years.

Modes of digitalization

If atrial fibrillation is associated with an excessively rapid ventricular response, producing actual or impending congestive heart failure, digitalization may be accomplished rapidly.

Intravenous digitalization may be carried out using digoxin, ouabain, or lanatoside C. Remember that intravenous digitalization is hazardous and be sure to observe the precautions listed in Chapter 19.

If the ventricular rate is not extremely rapid and the patient is not immediately threatened, oral digitalization may be completed in 24 hours and subsequent daily maintenance doses given.

If the ventricular rhythm is near the normal range and if treatment of the arrhythmia is not an emergency, the patient may even be digitalized on an outpatient basis using one of the "slow digitalization" schedules listed in Chapter 12.

Digitoxin or powdered digitalis leaf may also be used, but both have the inherent disadvantage of prolonged excretion compared to digoxin.

Remember two rules in digitalizing patients with atrial fibrillation!

1. Older patients will need much less digoxin than younger ones because of the poor renal excretion of the drug in the older age group.
2. Thyrotoxic patients will need a great deal more of any digitalis preparation to slow the ventricular rate to acceptable levels. Reserpine (0.1 mg three times a day) may be given in thyrotoxic patients while digitalization is being completed.

Chronic anticoagulant therapy

A patient with chronic atrial fibrillation and an enlarged left atrium runs a high risk of arterial embolism. Therefore, patients with *valvular heart disease, atrial enlargement,* and *chronic atrial fibrillation* who *cannot* undergo corrective surgery for some reason should be maintained on anticoagulant therapy permanently.

On the other hand, chronic atrial fibrillation associated with arteriosclerotic heart disease, *without* atrial enlargement, is not likely to produce arterial emboli. In this group of patients the risk of anticoagulant therapy is probably greater than the risk of emboli.

REFERENCES

Abildskov, J., Millar, K., and Burgess, M.: Atrial fibrillation, Am. J. Cardiol. **28**:263-267, 1971.
Bellet, S.: Essentials of cardiac arrhythmias, Philadelphia, 1972, W. B. Saunders Co.
Benchimol, A., Lowe, H., and Akre, P.: Cardiovascular response to exercise during atrial fibrillation and after conversion to sinus rhythm, Am. J. Cardiol. **16**:31-41, 1965.
Friedberg, H.: Atrial fibrillation and digitalis toxicity, Am. Heart J. **77**:429-430, 1969.
Hornsten, T., and Bruce, R.: Effects of atrial fibrillation on exercise performance in patients with cardiac disease, Circulation **37**:543-548, 1968.
Khaja, F., and Parker, J.: Hemodynamic effects of cardioversion in chronic atrial fibrillation, Arch. Intern. Med. **129**:433-440, 1972.
Peter, R., Gracey, J., and Beach, T.: A clinical profile of idiopathic atrial fibrillation: a functional disorder of atrial rhythm, Ann. Intern. Med. **68**:1288-1300, 1968.
Radford, M., and Evans, D.: Long-term results of DC reversion of atrial fibrillation, Brit. Heart J. **30**:91-96, 1968.
Urbach, J., Grauman, J., and Straus, S.: Effects of inspiration, expiration, and apnea upon pacemaking and block in atrial fibrillation, Circulation **42**:261-269, 1970.

10 Atrial flutter

Atrial flutter is a rapid, regular, continuous wave movement in the atria. This arrhythmia is considerably rarer than atrial fibrillation, although the causes are generally the same.

MECHANISM

The term "atrial flutter" describes the arrhythmia very well. To visualize atrial flutter, hold your clenched fists one above the other. The top fist represents the atria and the bottom fist represents the ventricles. Open and shut the top fist as rapidly and regularly as possible. This is approximately what a flutter movement looks like—a rapid, continuous "flapping" movement of the atria that is perfectly regular in timing and amplitude.

Now open and shut the bottom hand (the "ventricles") at a slower rate so that it contracts once to every four contractions of the "atria." This is the sequence of events in atrial flutter (Fig. 10-1).

Inspect Fig. 10-2. The mechanism is obvious. The large, perfectly regular, saw-toothed waves shown in the tracing correspond to the flutter waves traversing the atria. Place a pair of calipers on any two of the wave peaks and measure on through the strip. Note that the timing of these waves is perfectly regular and that the contour of all the flutter waves is identical. These two points are characteristic. There are four flutter waves for each ventricular response, hence this is called a 4:1 flutter. The reason for the disparity between the atrial and ventricular rates is simple. Since the atrial rate is about 300, all the atrial impulses cannot traverse the A-V node. Many of the impulses will find the node refractory from the passage of the previous impulse and thus will be blocked. Note that the peak of one flutter wave (f_4) is hidden by the QRS complex with which it coincides.

DIAGNOSIS

Bedside diagnosis of flutter is inaccurate and unsatisfactory for reasons that will be made clear in this chapter. *The diagnosis of flutter is based on recognition of flutter waves in one or more leads of the electrocardiogram* (Fig. 10-3, B). The ventricular rate is of no help. If the ratio of conduction from the atria to the ventricles is constant (2:1, for example), the ventricular rate will be regular. If the ratio of conduction changes from moment to moment (2:1 to 4:1 to 3:1), the ventricular rate will be completely irregular. The pulse then cannot be differentiated from that of atrial fibrillation.

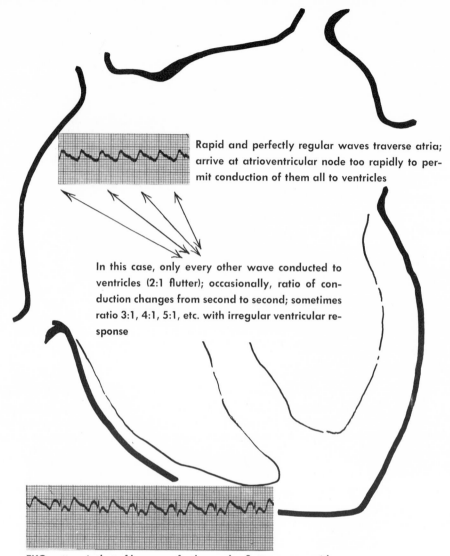

Rapid and perfectly regular waves traverse atria; arrive at atrioventricular node too rapidly to permit conduction of them all to ventricles

In this case, only every other wave conducted to ventricles (2:1 flutter); occasionally, ratio of conduction changes from second to second; sometimes ratio 3:1, 4:1, 5:1, etc. with irregular ventricular response

EKG pattern is that of large, perfectly regular flutter waves with ventricular complexes superimposed at intervals

Fig. 10-1. Atrial flutter.

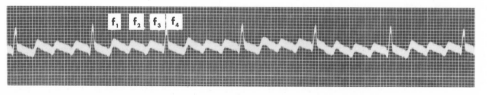

Fig. 10-2. Atrial flutter. The large saw-toothed atrial complexes are labeled *f*. This is a 4:1 flutter.

To diagnose flutter, the physician must learn to recognize flutter waves in the electrocardiogram. In Fig. 10-4, the ratio of conduction is 2:1. The flutter waves shown in this strip are more rounded on the top than those shown in Fig. 10-2. At the end of each wave, notice the sharp V formed by the junction with the upstroke that starts the next wave. *This is another characteristic finding.*

A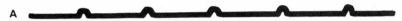

Normal P waves are separate with definite flat "quiet" period between waves—how P waves would look if there were no ventricular response

B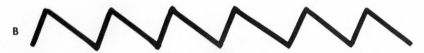

Flutter waves continuous: no quiet period; end of one down-stroke followed at once by next upstroke

C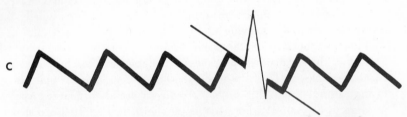

One can place ruler along flutter wave which starts just before ventricular complex and find end of flutter wave after ventricular complex, along same line

Fig. 10-3. Differentiation of flutter waves from normal sinus complexes.

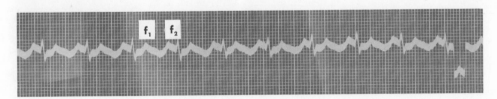

Fig. 10-4. Atrial flutter (2:1 ratio).

Observe that the flutter waves shown in Fig. 10-4, labeled f_2, seem to "pass through" the ventricular complex and come out on the other side. This is a very helpful diagnostic point (Fig. 10-3, C). You can place a ruler along a flutter wave that starts just before a ventricular complex and find the end of the flutter wave after the ventricular complex along the same line.

Take care! Flutter waves are not visible in every lead! Figs. 10-5 and 10-6 show leads I and II taken on the same patient at the same time. Lead I seems to indicate an atrial or nodal tachycardia. Only when you carefully inspect lead II do you see the characteristic flutter waves. It is often necessary to take all twelve standard leads plus extra precordial leads over the right precordium to find flutter waves. In the tracings shown in Fig. 10-5 a 2:1 ratio is illustrated. These flutter waves are narrower and steeper than those shown in Fig. 10-4. The V's formed by the final downstroke of one wave and the initial upstroke of the next are sharp and clear. One comes just before and one just after each ventricular complex.

Sometimes flutter waves are very wide. The contour of the upstroke or downstroke may show "humps," as may be seen in Fig. 10-7. The wave does not form a completely smooth saw tooth. The diagnostic points are as follows:

1. There is continuous atrial activity since the end of one wave is followed at once by the beginning of the next wave.
2. Each atrial wave looks exactly like every other atrial wave.
3. The timing of the atrial complexes is perfectly regular.
4. The V contour at the junction of the atrial waves is apparent.

The tracing shown in Fig. 10-8 presents a strong argument against bedside diagnosis. About one third of all patients with atrial flutter show irregular conduction to the ventricles. For instance, the ratio of conduction will vary from 2:1 to 4:1 to 3:1 in successive beats. As a result, the radial pulse will be completely irregular. In the electrocardiogram, however, the flutter waves are obvious. Flutter waves are supposed to be visible in the jugular veins on clinical inspection. Occasionally they are but not nearly often enough to provide a reliable diagnostic criterion.

Flutter or not? From the tracing shown in Fig. 10-9 you would suspect flutter because of the saw-tooth appearance of the complex seen between each pair of ventricular complexes. To make the diagnosis obvious in such patients, apply pressure to the carotid sinus. This is an exceedingly useful maneuver. Application of such pressure to the patient whose tracing is shown in Fig. 10-9 arrested the ventricular response, as shown in Fig. 10-10. The isolated flutter waves are now perfectly clear and the diagnosis is unmistakable.

In summary, atrial flutter is a rapid, regular, continuous wave movement in the atria. This wave movement may produce a regular or irregular ventricular response, depending on the ratio of conduction to the ventricles. Diagnosis depends on the

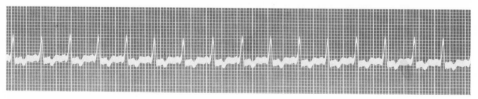

Fig. 10-5. Atrial flutter. In lead I shown here, it would be very difficult to diagnose flutter. (See Fig. 10-6.)

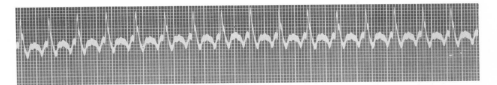

Fig. 10-6. Atrial flutter. Lead II on the same patient as in Fig. 10-5. Flutter waves are obvious in this lead.

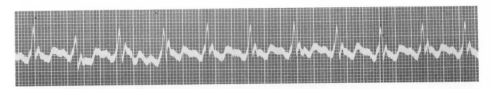

Fig. 10-7. Atrial flutter. Note the wide, notched character of the flutter waves.

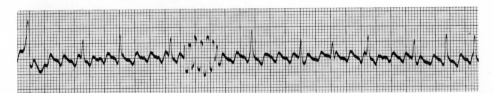

Fig. 10-8. Atrial flutter. The ratio of conduction to the ventricles changes from beat to beat so that the apical rate is completely irregular.

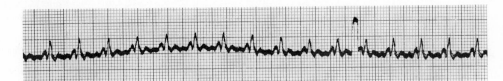

Fig. 10-9. Is this flutter? It would be difficult to be certain from inspection of this tracing. (See Fig. 10-10.)

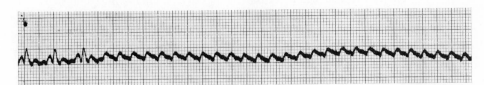

Fig. 10-10. Carotid sinus pressure halts the ventricular response after the third beat on the strip. Isolated, obvious flutter waves are recorded across the rest of the tracing. This is a very important diagnostic maneuver.

demonstration of flutter waves in one or more leads of the electrocardiogram. Flutter waves are continuous, regular, and identical.

CLINICAL MANIFESTATIONS

The onset of atrial flutter is abrupt and will usually produce symptoms of "pounding of the heart" or "palpitation." Dyspnea may be precipitated by the arrhythmia in a person who has some degree of organic heart disease. I have heard atrial flutter described as a "cold in the chest" by a patient who wished a telephone prescription to "clear the congestion."

Vagal stimulation produces a slowing of the ventricular rate in many patients with atrial flutter. This takes place because of an abrupt rise in the degree of block in the A-V node (that is, from 2:1 to 6:1 or 8:1). I have produced asystole that lasted for several seconds by using carotid sinus pressure on a patient with flutter. This gives an excellent electrocardiographic confirmation of the flutter, but in an elderly patient it may involve some risk.

Visible flutter waves are sometimes detectable in the jugular veins. They appear as very rapid "flickering" motions that will usually be more visible at one phase of respiration than another, depending upon the type of breathing and the patient's habitus. Flutter waves are sometimes absolutely not visible, even though a flutter may be shown to be present on the electrocardiogram. This physical finding, while of great interest, is not sufficiently reliable to establish or deny the diagnosis of atrial flutter.

TREATMENT

As in atrial fibrillation, there are two goals of treatment of atrial flutter:
1. Conversion of the atrial flutter to a normal sinus mechanism OR
2. Slowing of the ventricular rate to ensure optimal ventricular function
The rules about the treatment of atrial flutter can be stated very simply:
1. Use digitalis to produce a 3:1 or 4:1 ratio of conduction from atria to ventricles. This will practically always ensure a ventricular rate somewhere in the normal range and will often be lifesaving if the rapid rate and inefficient mechanism of flutter have led to congestive heart failure.
2. Convert the fibrillation to a sinus mechanism by quinidine or electroversion.
Atrial flutter is the indication par excellence for electroversion. There is an extremely high ratio of success, and the energy levels required for conversion are fantastically small. Shocks of 10 to 15 watt-seconds are usually successful in terminating a flutter and instituting normal sinus rhythm. If a patient has been in failure with a dilated atrium, it is probably well to digitalize first and produce maximum tissue oxygenation and minimal chamber dilation before attempting electroshock therapy.

Frequently, during digitalization the atrial flutter will spontaneously convert to atrial fibrillation. At this time, digitalis should be withheld and a normal sinus rhythm will often spontaneously follow. If for some reason electroshock is not available, quinidine may be used to convert the flutter directly to a sinus mechanism. Quinidine, 100 mg hourly or 200 mg every 2 hours, may be given for 12 hours, with careful observation for toxic effects. After the first 12 hours, dosage must be regulated by the patient's response and by the presence or absence of side effects. Quinidine is very efficient in converting flutter to normal sinus rhythm, but it does not compare with electroshock for efficacy or safety.

WARNING: When quinidine is used a curious and possibly disastrous effect may follow. The quinidine actually slows the flutter waves so that they are wider on the electrocardiogram. When this slowing has progressed sufficiently, each flutter wave may come through and stimulate the ventricles with a 1:1 ratio of flutter waves to ventricular response. The ventricles will then begin beating at a rate of 300 per minute in an effort to "keep up" with the fluttering atria. In an elderly or seriously ill patient, this may be catastrophic.

To avoid this dangerous complication, *always digitalize first* and then employ quinidine if necessary.

REFERENCES

Agarwal, B. L., and others: Atrial flutter: a rare manifestation of digitalis intoxication, Brit. Heart J. **34**:392-395, 1972.

Chung, E. K.: Principles of cardiac arrhythmias, Baltimore, 1971, The Williams & Wilkins Co.

Harvey, R., and others: Cardiocirculatory performance in atrial flutter, Circulation **12**:507-519, 1955.

Katz, L., and Pick, A.: Clinical electrocardiography: Part I. The arrhythmias, Philadelphia, 1956, Lea & Febiger.

Lau, S., and others: A study of atrioventricular conduction in atrial fibrillation and flutter in man using His bundle recordings, Circulation **40**:71-78, 1969.

Rosner, S.: Atrial tachysystole with block, Circulation **29**:614-621, 1964.

Scherf, D.: The mechanism of flutter and fibrillation, Am. Heart J. **71**:273-288, 1966.

Wellens, H., and others: Epicardial excitation of the atria in a patient with atrial flutter, Brit. Heart J. **33**:233-237, 1971.

11 Problems, practice, and reinforcement: 2

PROBLEM 1: The tracing is recorded in a comatose patient seen in the emergency room following an accident. The patient has been taking "some kind of heart medicine" but the exact type is unknown (Fig. 11-1).

QUESTIONS:

1. Basic rhythm?
2. State of conductivity in the A-V tissue?
3. Management?

ANSWERS:

1. The basic rhythm is atrial fibrillation with moderately coarse fibrillary waves. Note the irregular spacing of the ventricular complexes.
2. There must be some kind of delay in A-V conduction because of the slow ventricular rate with the occasional long pauses in A-V conduction of $1\frac{1}{2}$ seconds or more. When atrial fibrillary complexes bombard the A-V conducting tissues at a rate of 400 a minute or more, a healthy A-V conducting system should produce a very rapid ventricular rate. With a ventricular response as slow as this, some degree of A-V block must be present. The block cannot be complete, however, because the ventricular rhythm is irregular, which means the ventricles are responding to the fibrillating atria.
3. Since the exact type of heart medication is unknown, it must be assumed that digitalis may be responsible for the delay in A-V conduction. No further digitalis preparations should be administered until the ventricular rate is in the normal range.

PROBLEM 2: A patient telephones you describing a "full feeling in his chest" that he attributes to a cold. (This is exactly what the patient described in this case.) Examination at your office reveals the electrocardiogram shown here. On the right side of the strip, carotid sinus pressure was applied (Fig. 11-2).

QUESTIONS:

1. Rhythm?
2. Unusual feature?
3. Reason for symptoms?
4. Treatment?

ANSWERS:

1. Atrial flutter with 2:1 A-V conduction is present on the left-hand side of the strip. During carotid sinus pressure, on the right-hand side of the strip, there is complete interruption of A-V conduction—there are flutter waves without any ventricular response.

2. The unusual feature is the relatively slow rate of the flutter waves—about 187. Atrial flutter is more commonly in the range of 280 to 300. The characteristic shape of the flutter waves here leaves no doubt about the diagnosis.

3. Almost any patient will describe some symptoms at the onset of flutter; these symptoms may be minor and baffling to the clinician, and they certainly underline the dictum: "Never treat a patient you haven't seen!"

4. Digitalize until the atrial waves are conducted to the ventricles with a 3:1 or 4:1 ratio and then convert to sinus rhythm with quinidine or electroversion. After digitalization the flutter may convert to fibrillation and then go on to a normal sinus rhythm spontaneously.

PROBLEM 3: A patient in the coronary care unit with an anterior myocardial infarct has had first-degree A-V block with the P-R interval of .26 second. The pause illustrated in the strip appears on the oscilloscope several times each minute (Fig. 11-3).

QUESTIONS:
1. Cause of pause?
2. Significance?
3. Action taken?

ANSWERS:
1. The cause of the pause here is a Mobitz Type 2 block. The P waves are in-

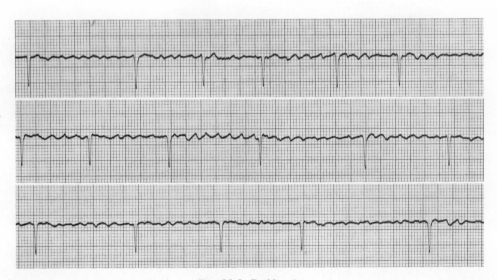

Fig. 11-1. Problem 1.

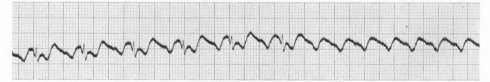

Fig. 11-2. Problem 2.

verted, which is often true in a monitor lead with eccentric placement of electrodes on the chest. The P-R interval is prolonged but fixed in the first two beats on this strip. The third P wave is a normal sinus P wave arriving at exactly the normal interval, but it is not conducted to the ventricles. Blocking of an occasional sinus P wave as illustrated here is characteristic of Mobitz Type 2 block. Note that the P-R interval in the conducted beats is constant, except for the first beat after the blocked P wave. Here the P-R interval is very slightly shorter than in the other beats. This, too, is a common finding in Mobitz Type 2 block.

2. Appearance of Mobitz Type 2 block instantly alerts the clinician to the possibility of a complete standstill. Mobitz Type 2 block is an ominous phenomenon and instantly increases the calculated risk. Second-degree block appearing in the presence of an anterior myocardial infarct implies a very high risk in any case.

3. Appearance of Mobitz Type 2 block in the course of a myocardial infarct is an indication for prompt insertion of a pacing catheter to the right ventricle with the pacemaker set on "Standby."

PROBLEM 4: A 65-year-old patient without previous history of cardiac disease complains of a "rapid, pounding sensation in his chest." The rhythm illustrated is detected at the time of examination (Fig. 11-4).

QUESTIONS:
1. Rhythm?
2. Significance?
3. Treatment?
4. Probable cause?

ANSWERS:
1. Atrial fibrillation with rapid ventricular response is demonstrated. There is one ventricular ectopic beat (first beat in this strip). Note the absence of P waves and the total irregularity of the ventricular rhythm.

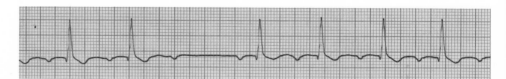

Fig. 11-3. Problem 3.

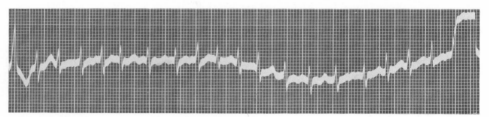

Fig. 11-4. Problem 4.

2. This rapid, inefficient ventricular rate and rhythm will soon produce congestive heart failure if allowed to persist. Prompt slowing of the ventricular rate with digitalis is indicated.

3. Treatment consists of rapid digitalization, intravenously or orally, the route depending on the clinical estimate of the urgency of the situation.

4. In an elderly patient without previous history of heart disease, it is likely that arteriosclerotic heart disease is the cause of the arrhythmia. *It is very important to rule out a "silent" myocardial infarct, which is often heralded by the onset of atrial fibrillation.*

PROBLEM 5: A patient with an anterior myocardial infarct who has had a normal sinus rhythm abruptly changes to the pattern shown on these strips (Fig. 11-5).

QUESTIONS:

1. Basic rhythm?
2. Location of pacemaker responsible for ventricular rhythm?
3. Treatment?
4. Prognosis?

ANSWERS:

1. The strips show complete heart block. Notice the relatively rapid atrial rhythm (125) with a much slower, completely independent ventricular rhythm. Remember the axiom: *In differentiating types of A-V block, a changing P-R interval with a regular ventricular rhythm almost always means complete heart block.*

2. The QRS complexes are wide; it is likely, therefore, that the pacemaker driving the ventricles and supporting life is located below the bifurcation of the bundle branches—that is, this is a true idioventricular rhythm. It is remotely possible that a junctional rhythm with bundle branch block could be responsible for these wide pacemakers, but this is not likely. Therefore, the diagnosis is complete A-V block, probably caused by bilateral bundle branch block.

3. Treatment consists of prompt insertion of a transvenous pacing catheter into the right ventricle.

4. Complete A-V block caused by bilateral bundle branch block is a very grave sign. In the presence of an anterior myocardial infarct, this implies an 85%

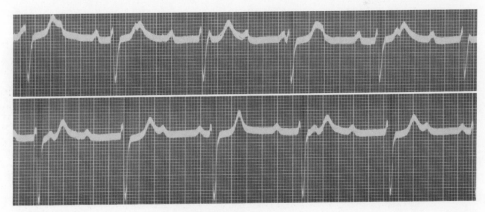

Fig. 11-5. Problem 5.

mortality, since it is likely that the left anterior descending branch of the left coronary artery has been occluded near its origin. The situation is desperate, and the most extreme measures are justified.

PROBLEM 6: The rhythm illustrated here is detected in a patient with chronic atrial fibrillation who has been taking digitalis for several years (Fig. 11-6).

QUESTIONS:

1. Rhythm?
2. Proof of diagnosis?
3. Significance?
4. Treatment?

ANSWERS:

1. Basic rhythm is atrial fibrillation interrupted by a number of wide ventricular complexes representing ventricular ectopic beats.
2. The wide complexes *might* be ventricular ectopic beats or they might be aberrantly conducted supraventricular beats from the fibrillating atria. The proof in such a problem lies in the detection of fusion beats. Compare the sixth beat with others in the tracing. The sixth beat is wide (.12 second), as is the thirteenth. The fifteenth and seventeenth beats are *intermediate* in form and width between the two widest beats and the narrow supraventricular complexes in the rest of the tracing and hence represent *fusion* beats. The conclusion is that the wide complexes are in fact ventricular ectopic beats. Note the fifteenth beat, which represents a type of fusion in which the supraventricular impulse has penetrated deeply across the ventricles before meeting the impulse from the ectopic ventricular focus, producing a QRS complex only slightly different from normal. Fusion beats are common when ventricular ectopic beats interrupt atrial fibrillation.
3. Detection of ventricular beats in the presence of atrial fibrillation is particularly important, since repetitive ventricular ectopic firing is a common and ominous sign of digitalis toxicity.
4. Stop digitalis. If repetive ventricular ectopic firing is a problem, administer Dilantin. (See Chapter 12.)

PROBLEM 7: A 68-year-old patient with mild essential hypertension and some evidence of diffuse arteriosclerosis describes brief paroxysms of "pounding of the heart" accompanied by a feeling of breathlessness. These are not related to exercise and seem to appear spontaneously without any obvious inciting cause. The tracing is recorded during one of these paroxysms (Fig. 11-7).

QUESTIONS:

1. What is the rhythm?
2. Treatment?
3. Significance?

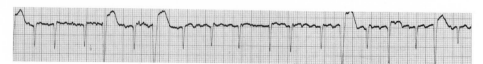

Fig. 11-6. Problem 6.

ANSWERS:

1. In the left-hand part of the top strip a search for the P waves, which should be the first part of analysis of any arrhythmia, reveals a P wave followed at a normal conducting distance by a ventricular complex in the fourth beat. The ventricular complex is wide (.12 second), indicating some type of intraventricular block. The first two ventricular complexes on this strip are wide and have a different shape from the fourth beat. These beats are not preceded by P waves and hence are probably ventricular ectopic beats. The third beat is clearly a fusion beat, with a P wave a short distance ahead of an "intermediate" ventricular complex, which is similar in shape to the first two beats but is narrower. The conclusion so far, therefore, is a normal sinus rhythm with intraventricular block, two ventricular ectopic beats, and one fusion beat. The fifth beat seems to be an ectopic beat from still another focus; this may be a junctional beat with aberrant conduction or it might be a ventricular ectopic beat. The sixth beat is preceded by a P wave at a normal conducting distance; the conclusion is that this is another normally conducted sinus beat. Following this, P waves disappear and a series of rapid, saw-toothed atrial complexes are seen, appearing at a rate of 188 per minute. The conclusion is that these waves probably represent atrial flutter. With the first three ventricular complexes following the onset of the flutter there is a 2:1 ratio of flutter waves to ventricular complexes. Between the third and fourth ventricular responses after the onset of flutter there are four flutter waves—the ratio of conduction from atria to ventricles suddenly varies. Through the rest of the top strip a 2:1 ratio continues. Between the second and third ventricular responses on the bottom strip, the ratio of flutter wave to ventricular response is seen to shift from 2:1 to 3:1.

   NOTE: The distance from flutter wave to ventricular response is always shorter with a high ratio of flutter waves to ventricular complexes (3:1 or 4:1) than it is with a 2:1 ratio. Notice in the period of 4:1 conduction in the top strip that the distance from the flutter wave to the ventricular complex that terminates this ratio is .14 second. The distance from flutter wave to ventricular complex when the ratio is 2:1 is approximately .16 or .17 second. Again, in the bottom strip when the ratio shifts from 2:1 to 3:1, the distance from flutter wave shortens to about .14 second. The answer is simple: the

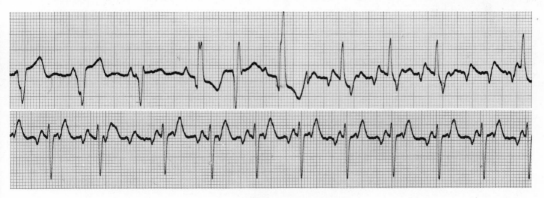

Fig. 11-7. Problem 7.

longer the period without conduction to the ventricles, the longer the A-V conducting tissues have to "rest" and attain maximum efficiency on the next transmission.

2. This patient presents several problems: paroxysmal atrial flutter and ventricular ectopic firing. If the patient is given only digitalis to control the flutter, the ventricular ectopic foci may become dangerously irritable and sustained ventricular ectopic rhythms may result. On the other hand, if quinidine is given, there is a danger that the flutter may turn to a 1:1 ratio with a very rapid ventricular response. This case would be best treated by simultaneous use of digitalis and quinidine. Since this, presumably, would be carried out on an outpatient basis and since there would be no immediate threat to life, oral use of both agents with one of the slower digitalizing schedules and a moderate level of quinidine (200 mg three or four times a day) would be indicated.

3. In an older patient with evidence of arteriosclerotic heart disease, paroxysmal arrhythmias like these are to be regarded with great suspicion, since their appearance may be a consequence of an undetected process in the myocardium. Besides controlling the arrhythmia, a thorough investigation for associated myocardial ischemic disease should be carried out. Again, in a patient of this category, this kind of paroxysmal arrhythmia may result in transient blunting of the sensorium or complete loss of consciousness, which might present real hazards in such activities as driving a car. Until the arrhythmia is brought under control, the patient's activities should probably be rather severely limited.

PROBLEM 8: A patient who has been taking 0.25 mg of digoxin daily for rheumatic valvular disease presents himself at the office stating that he is "feeling worse and more out of breath." His digitalis had been increased by another physician

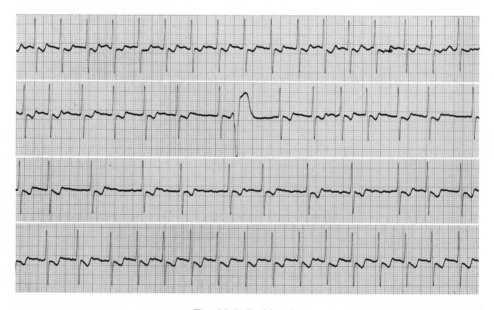

Fig. 11-8. Problem 8.

to 0.25 mg twice a day about a week prior to this visit. The comment by the referring physician is that "the more digitalis I give him, the worse this man seems to get" (Fig. 11-8).

QUESTIONS:

1. Basic rhythm?
2. Complication?
3. Cause?
4. Prognosis?
5. Treatment?

ANSWERS:

1. Basic rhythm is atrial fibrillation, as noted in the middle two strips. One ventricular ectopic beat is present.
2. The top and bottom strips of this tracing show an almost perfectly regular rhythm with narrow ventricular complexes, indicating a supraventricular origin. No P waves are visible. Except for a slight change in interval between the first and second and third and fourth complexes in the bottom strip, the rhythm is perfectly regular and the rate is much more rapid than the ventricular rate during the period of atrial fibrillation (100, as compared to approximately 70). *Diagnosis, therefore, is A-V junctional rhythm (accelerated A-V junctional rhythm) interrupting atrial fibrillation.*
3. Digitalis toxicity is a very common cause of this phenomenon. The combination of increased block in the A-V node with some toxic acceleration of a junctional pacemaker produces this intermittent regular rhythm interrupting the atrial fibrillation.
4. Appearance of an ectopic regular rhythm interrupting atrial fibrillation is a grave sign of digitalis toxicity. Digitalis should be stopped at once. Further administration of digitalis at this point might well threaten life.
5. Withdraw digitalis. Suppressive drugs will serve little or no useful purpose here. General supportive measures may be necessary if signs of failure appear, but no other specific intervention is indicated.

PROBLEM 9: A 45-year-old patient with a history of coronary artery disease, angina pectoris, and intermittent mild congestive heart failure who has been taking digitalis presents at the emergency room with what is described as a "rapid, irregular pulse, suggestive of atrial fibrillation." The electrocardiogram is recorded here (Fig. 11-9).

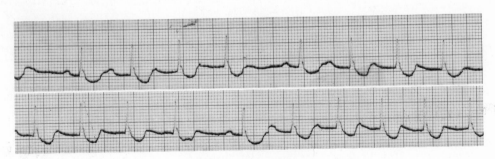

Fig. 11-9. Problem 9.

QUESTIONS:

1. Basic rhythm?
2. Possible causes?
3. Treatment?

ANSWERS:

1. The rhythm is a Wenckebach type of heart block. A P wave is clearly seen preceding the first beat in the upper strip. The first P-R interval is about .20 second, the second P-R interval lengthens to approximately .31 second, and the next two P-R intervals become longer, but exact measurement is not possible because the P wave "moves into" the T wave of the preceding beat. The fifth P wave of this cycle is blocked, and there is a pause followed by a beat with a short P-R interval. Note that the Wenckebach cycles in the top strip run four conducted beats before the fifth P wave is blocked, while in the bottom strip there are five and six P waves conducted, respectively, in the two Wenckebach cycles, before a P wave is finally blocked.

2. Since the Wenckebach type of A-V block is commonly caused by disease of the A-V node, it is likely that digitalis toxicity is the cause of the A-V block. It is also possible that a myocardial ischemic episode involving the septal tissues might be the cause. Associated symptoms and laboratory studies should be evaluated carefully with these two possibilities in mind. The "drooping" S-T segments strongly suggest digitalis effect, but this does not necessarily mean that the digitalis is the actual cause of the Wenckebach phenomenon.

3. First, stop digitalis. Second, observe carefully for change in block on withdrawal of digitalis effect.

PROBLEM 10: A patient with hypertensive heart disease and a history of angina pectoris is seen in the coronary care unit describing abrupt onset of pounding rapid action of the heart and very difficult breathing. Physical examination reveals that the patient is obviously in congestive heart failure. A rapid regular pulse is noted, except for some brief interludes when a slow pulse is detected for a few seconds. The electrocardiogram appears here (Fig. 11-10).

QUESTIONS:

1. Rhythm?
2. Associated finding?
3. Treatment?

ANSWERS:

1. From leads I, II, and III alone it would not be possible to diagnose this rhythm. For the most part, the rhythm is perfectly regular in these leads, with a rate of slightly under 150. The QRS complexes are wide (.16 second) and no P waves are noted. The possibility of *paroxysmal ventricular tachycardia* must therefore be considered. The abrupt change in rate in V_1 gives a clue to the answer; here the rate suddenly drops from 150 to 75. Inspection of aV_F reveals another clue. Note the jagged, almost saw-toothed waves between the QRS complexes. The only rhythm in which the ventricular rate will suddenly drop by half and then resume its original rate is atrial flutter. The ratio of conduction suddenly switches from 2:1 to 4:1; since the atrial flutter rate is 300, this produces a drop in ventricular response from 150 to 75. The flutter waves noted in lead aV_F further confirm this diagnosis. This peculiar phenomenon of "halving" the ventricular rate is characteristic

of flutter; the diagnosis should always be suspected when this is seen. Close inspection of lead V_1 reveals small, notched atrial complexes between the ventricular complexes. The flutter waves are seen here only in aV_F. Carotid sinus pressure, with recording of aV_F, would doubtless make the diagnosis obvious.

2. With the conclusion that atrial flutter is the mechanism and that the ventricular complexes represent a response to the flutter, the diagnosis of bundle branch block is also established. This is a right bundle branch block, based on the configuration of lead V_1.

3. This should be treated as any flutter, with initial digitalis and subsequent electroversion. If the patient is in critical condition and termination of the rhythm seems urgent, electroversion might be considered early in the course of treatment.

PROBLEM 11: A patient presents in the emergency room with substernal oppression, low blood pressure, and a weak, slow pulse. The rhythm illustrated here appears on the oscilloscope (Fig. 11-11).

QUESTIONS:

1. Basic rhythm?
2. Treatment?

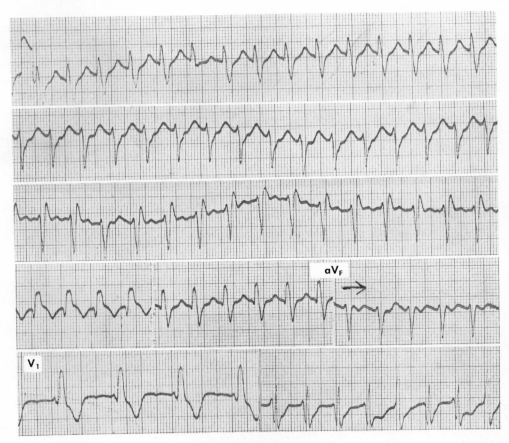

Fig. 11-10. Problem 10.

3. Assuming myocardial infarction, what does this rhythm tell about the prognosis?

ANSWERS:

1. A sinus rhythm with a high degree of A-V block is present. In the first beat in the top strip a P wave is followed by a ventricular complex at a normal interval. The second P wave is followed, after a prolonged P-R interval (.24 second), by a wide QRS. The third complex again consists of a prolonged P-R interval (.26 second) with a slightly wider QRS complex. The fourth complex consists of a wide, bizarre QRS complex without an apparent P wave. The abrupt deflection in the baseline preceding the ventricular complex here may be an artifact. With the fifth beat, there is again a normal P-R relationship. The next three ventricular complexes are somewhat wider than the normal ventricular complex of the fifth beat and are not preceded at a "normal conducting distance" by a P wave. In the ninth beat there is a slightly prolonged P-R interval with a normal ventricular complex, followed by a blocked P wave. The tenth ventricular complex seems to represent normal conduction from atria to ventricles. In the bottom strip two conducted beats are followed by a blocked P wave, which is followed in turn by a conducted beat (the third beat on the bottom strip), followed again by a blocked P wave, the whole strip being terminated by three wide beats with no relationship to P waves. The conclusion, therefore, is that the wide beats appearing intermittently are ventricular escape beats—short runs of an idioventricular rhythm. It is obvious from inspection of the last three ventricular complexes in the bottom strip and the sixth, seventh, and eighth complexes in the top strip that these are indeed ventricular ectopic beats forming an idioventricular rhythm, since they are not preceded by P waves. The same is doubtless true of the second, third, and fourth beats, the relation to the P waves probably being coincidental.

2. Treatment consists of *prompt* insertion of a pacing electrode into the right ventricle. Atropine might be administered for any possible antivagal effect, with possible diminution of the degree of A-V block.

3. If the patient has an anterior myocardial infarct, the appearance of a high degree of block indicates an extremely grave prognosis with an 85% mortality. With an inferior myocardial infarct, prognosis is much less serious, with a maximum mortality between 30% and 36%. Regardless of location of the infarct, with this degree of block a pacing catheter should be inserted and tested for performance.

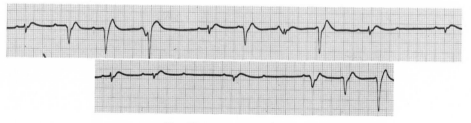

Fig. 11-11. Problem 11.

PROBLEM 12: A patient with an anterior myocardial infarct has had first-degree A-V block with a P-R interval of .25 second. The mean frontal plane axis of the electrocardiogram has been +30 degrees. The patient describes some precordial oppression, together with a feeling of weakness. The electrocardiogram recorded immediately thereafter shows this configuration (leads are limb leads I, II, and III, top to bottom) (Fig. 11-12).

QUESTIONS:

1. What is the present diagnosis?
2. In view of the previous normal frontal plane axis, what pathologic event has taken place?
3. What prognostic significance does this have, and what steps should be taken?

ANSWERS:

1. Pathologic left axis is present (approximately −45 degrees). The QRS complexes are slightly widened (.11 second) and there is counterclockwise rotation of the electrocardiographic force in the frontal plane.
2. With a shift from an axis of +30 degrees to −45 degrees, together with the other changes noted, it is clear that the anterior-superior fascicle of the left bundle branch is no longer conducting. This finding, together with the patient's symptoms, indicates acute ischemic change in the septum.
3. When a myocardial infarct first produces a prolonged P-R interval and then produces evidence of blocking of one fascicle of the left bundle branch, the clinician must be alert for a progressive ischemic process that may completely interrupt A-V conduction. Particular attention should now be paid to lead V_1 for evidence of delay in right bundle branch. If these changes appeared in rapid sequence it might be well to have a transvenous pacing catheter in the right ventricle on standby, since interruption of conduction through the remaining fascicles might take place very suddenly, with production of ventricular standstill.

PROBLEM 13: A patient with acute rheumatic carditis who has previously had a slightly prolonged P-R interval manifests the arrhythmia shown here (Fig. 11-13).

QUESTIONS:

1. Type of block?

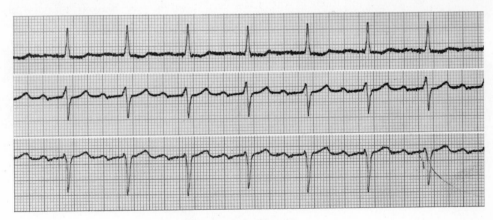

Fig. 11-12. Problem 12.

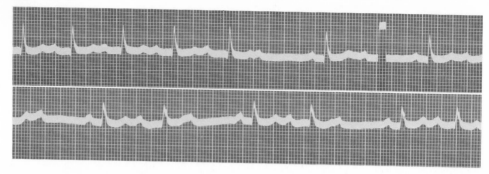

Fig. 11-13. Problem 13.

2. Possible localization of block anatomically?

ANSWERS:

1. The first five beats on the top strip show a gradual prolongation of P-R interval until the sixth P wave is blocked. In other words, a typical Wenckebach phenomenon is present. In the remainder of the strip a 2:1 block is noted (ignore the standardizing signal between the sixth and seventh ventricular complexes). At the beginning of the bottom strip a 2:1 block is still present, but this shifts to a Wenckebach relationship, with every third P wave being blocked. This strip emphasizes several phenomena about second-degree block of the Wenckebach type. First, the cycle length may vary a great deal. In the top strip there are five conducted beats before a P wave is blocked, whereas in the bottom strip every third P wave is blocked. Second, 2:1 block is often found, varying with Wenckebach conduction; in these cases, the 2:1 block is simply another form of Wenckebach—that is, it may be thought of as a "two-beat" Wenckebach phenomenon. Third, 3:2 A-V conduction—conduction of two P waves with blocking of the third—gives rise to a bigeminal pulse, which would be very difficult to distinguish at the bedside from a simple bigeminy produced by a premature beat appearing every other beat.

2. The Wenckebach type of A-V block is much more commonly found in the A-V node than in the bundle branch system. In the presence of inflammatory carditis, such as rheumatic carditis, it is very unlikely that the block will become a dangerous process per se. The chief interest for the clinician is that the progression of A-V block provides some idea of the course of the myocarditis.

Part III
COMPLEX ARRHYTHMIAS

Before completing this section of the book, the student should take a few moments for critical self-evaluation. The basic skills that he should have acquired at this point include:

1. Clinical and electrocardiographic diagnosis of:
    a. Sinus rhythms
    b. Ectopic firing, single and sustained
    c. Atrioventricular block
    d. Intraventricular block
    e. Atrial flutter and fibrillation
2. Ability to recognize aberration and fusion and to evaluate these phenomena
3. Familiarization with the major prognostic and therapeutic implications of all the arrhythmias

If these subjects are not reasonably familiar, *go back and review!* It is very easy to make a complete muddle of the complex arrhythmias because the simple arrhythmias are not really understood.

The complex cardiac arrhythmias represent various combinations of the basic disorders of rhythm. As a class, the complex arrhythmias often challenge the clinician with life-and-death decisions. Probably the most common complex arrhythmias are those produced by digitalis toxicity. This class of arrhythmia has become many times more common since the introduction of powerful diuretics with their potassium-wasting effect. The section on complex arrhythmias, therefore, begins with a consideration of these dangerous disorders of rhythm.

12 Digitalis-induced arrhythmias

Toxic levels of digitalis have two pathologic effects on cardiac conducting tissues that may be noted separately or in combination. These are:

1. Excessive vagal stimulation, which produces delay in conduction through the A-V node (A-V block) (This same vagal effect may also depress the rate of discharge of the S-A node.)
2. Excessive stimulation or "acceleration" of ectopic pacemakers anywhere in the heart (Fig. 12-1)

In other words, the toxic effects of digitalis on the conducting system will include:

1. A-V block of any degree
2. Depression of the S-A node
3. Ectopic firing, single or sustained, from any focus

These disorders of rhythm appearing *singly* are "simple" arrhythmias. As the student already knows, they may have many causes—they are not, per se, evidence of digitalis toxicity. On the other hand, the appearance of any one of these types of arrhythmia in a patient receiving digitalis should at once alert the clinician to the possibility of digitalis toxicity. Some simple rules follow.

1. When A-V block of any degree appears in the course of digitalis therapy it must be assumed that digitalis effect is producing the A-V nodal delay. Minimal first-degree A-V block might be called "digitalis effect" rather than "digitalis toxicity," and it is not necessarily grounds for discontinuing the drug. Any prolongation of the P-R interval, however, should alert the physician to the possibility of digitalis toxicity with progressive A-V block: the most careful observation is required. Severe first-degree A-V block, or any type of second or third-degree A-V block, in a patient receiving digitalis almost always requires that the drug be discontinued.

2. Multiple premature beats from any site in the heart appearing in a digitalized patient should be regarded as evidence of digitalis toxicity. Multiple ventricular ectopic beats are the most common arrhythmia produced by digitalis intoxication and are frequently an indication to stop the drug. The dangers of ectopic beats must be balanced against the needs of the patient—the decision to discontinue digitalis is not always a simple one.

3. Paroxysmal tachycardia of any type appearing in a digitalized patient should be regarded as a digitalis-induced arrhythmia until proved otherwise. Withdrawal of the drug should be the first step in treatment.

4. Accelerated junctional or ventricular rhythms (idiojunctional or idioventricular rhythms in the range of 90 to 110) are commonly evidence of digitalis

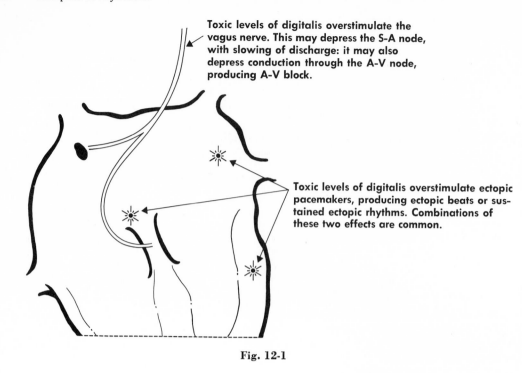

Toxic levels of digitalis overstimulate the vagus nerve. This may depress the S-A node, with slowing of discharge: it may also depress conduction through the A-V node, producing A-V block.

Toxic levels of digitalis overstimulate ectopic pacemakers, producing ectopic beats or sustained ectopic rhythms. Combinations of these two effects are common.

Fig. 12-1

toxicity. Again, the appearance of such rhythms is usually an indication for stopping digitalis.

The disorders of rhythm listed here are simple arrhythmias and should not present any diagnostic problems to the clinician at this point. It is necessary only to reemphasize the need for constant alertness on the part of the clinician for the appearance of any of these disorders of rhythm in a patient receiving digitalis.

COMPLEX ARRHYTHMIAS CAUSED BY DIGITALIS TOXICITY

Often the two basic toxic mechanisms of digitalis will combine to produce arrhythmias. There will be a combination of vagal effect (A-V block or S-A depression) and ectopic acceleration effect, with discharge of ectopic pacemakers. The simplest illustration of this combined effect is listed here as the first of the complex digitalis-toxic arrhythmias.

Delay or block of premature atrial beats

Toxic levels of digitalis often produce ectopic atrial beats. At the same time, the excessive vagal effect of the digitalis may slow conduction through the A-V node. Premature atrial beats, with delayed or blocked A-V nodal conduction, are a common sign of digitalis toxicity and may provide the earliest warning to the cardiologist.

Fig. 12-2 illustrates this phenomenon. There are many premature atrial beats in this strip. Most of the premature atrial beats manifest prolonged P-R intervals. (Note the premature atrial beats following the first, fourth, sixth, and ninth ventricular complexes.) *The fact that an atrial beat is ectopic does not explain a prolonged P-R interval. The upper limits of normal A-V conduction apply to ectopic atrial*

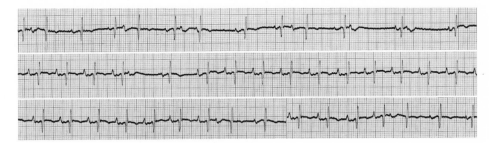

Fig. 12-2. Repeated atrial ectopic firing with varying degrees of A-V block (see text).

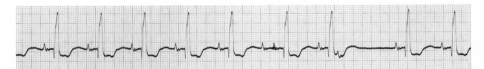

Fig. 12-3. Blocked premature atrial beat. The P wave following the seventh ventricular complex is premature—note that it is *not* conducted to the ventricles. (The sixth P wave actually was conducted to the ventricles; the dark, smudged area in the baseline after this P wave simply indicates the point at which the monitor was turned off.)

beats as well as to sinus beats, that is, a P-R interval of not more than .20 second. The appearance of such beats in a digitalized patient should make the clinician suspicious of digitalis toxicity.

Following the eleventh ventricular complex in this strip there is a completely blocked premature atrial beat. Note the P wave immediately following the QRS complex. There is also a blocked premature atrial beat after the twelfth ventricular complex; in this case, the P wave is so close to the preceding QRS that it is difficult to see.

In the second strip the fifth P wave is blocked; the beat that follows it seems to be an atrial escape beat from another ectopic focus, and normal sinus rhythm is then maintained. Note that the evidence of digitalis toxicity comes and goes in these two strips. If one were to look only at the right-hand side of the second strip, there would be no reason to suspect excessive digitalis effect.

Figs. 12-3 to 12-5 illustrate the same phenomenon of blocking or delay of conduction of ectopic atrial beats. Study the legends under these figures carefully. The ability to recognize this early and sometimes subtle manifestation of digitalis toxicity may be lifesaving.

Paroxysmal atrial tachycardia with atrioventricular block

Carry the complex arrhythmia just illustrated one step further. Imagine that the ectopic atrial focus goes on firing rapidly and regularly, forming a paroxysm of atrial tachycardia. Combine this atrial tachycardia with any degree of block in the A-V node and the result is a very common and a very dangerous arrhythmia *usually caused by physicians!*

Three statements about paroxysmal atrial tachycardia with A-V block should be burned deep in the mind of every physician who cares for cardiac patients:

1. Three quarters of all cases of paroxysmal atrial tachycardia with A-V block are caused by digitalis toxicity associated with an abnormally low serum potassium. This combination is usually the result of diuretic medication.

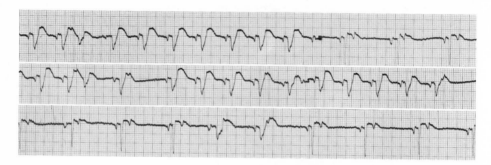

Fig. 12-4. Repeated blocking of premature atrial beats. On the right-hand side of the top strip note that each sinus beat is followed by a premature atrial beat that is blocked. The same phenomenon is repeated throughout the tracing. A blocked premature atrial beat is noted after the fourth ventricular complex in the second strip and after most of the ventricular complexes in the lower strip. (Note the rate-dependent bundle branch block.)

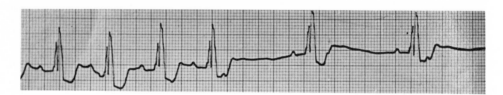

Fig. 12-5. Premature atrial beats appear on the right-hand side of this strip. Following the fourth ventricular complex, a premature atrial beat appears; this is blocked. Similar premature beats follow the fifth and sixth ventricular complexes, and they too are blocked. On the right-hand side of the strip, note the extremely slow ventricular rate as a consequence of blocking of the premature atrial beats.

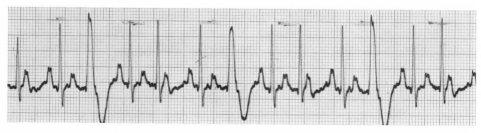

Fig. 12-6. Paroxysmal atrial tachycardia with A-V block. Atrial rhythm is rapid (188) and regular. Numerous ventricular ectopic beats are present. When not interrupted by the ventricular premature beats, a recurrent Wenckebach type of block is noted. (The first beat following the ventricular premature beat has a short P-R interval [.13 second]; the second beat in the sequence has a P-R of .18 second, and the third P wave is blocked. Thus, except for the irregularity produced by ventricular ectopic firing, a 3:2 Wenckebach cycle is noted throughout the tracing.) Ventricular ectopic firing is of course another manifestation of digitalis toxicity. The combination of these two digitalis-toxic arrhythmias is extremely dangerous.

2. Paroxysmal atrial tachycardia with A-V block may produce any variation of ventricular rhythm imaginable. The rhythm of the ventricles may be slow, rapid, regular, or irregular. "Bedside" or "clinical" diagnosis of paroxysmal atrial tachycardia with A-V block should never enter anyone's mind—it really isn't possible.

3. The treatment of digitalis-induced paroxysmal atrial tachycardia with A-V block is replacement of potassium. The wrong treatment—more digitalis—will produce a 36% mortality. *Paroxysmal atrial tachycardia with A-V block is a dangerous arrhythmia.*

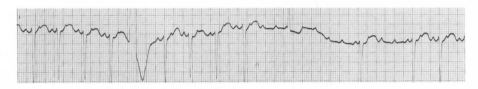

Fig. 12-7. Paroxysmal atrial tachycardia with block, with one ventricular ectopic beat and one fusion beat (the tenth complex on the tracing). The pause in the ventricular response was produced by carotid sinus pressure; notice how this maneuver reveals the rapid, regular, atrial mechanism with a rate of approximately 214. From the left-hand side of this strip alone it would be very difficult to make the diagnosis. Carotid sinus pressure is exceedingly useful in difficult cases of paroxysmal atrial tachycardia with block.

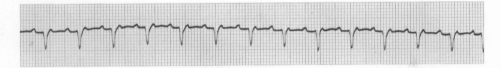

Fig. 12-8. 2:1 paroxysmal atrial tachycardia with A-V block. The blocked P in each cycle forms a small "hump" that looks like an R wave in the terminal portion of each ventricular complex. Atrial rate is 250.

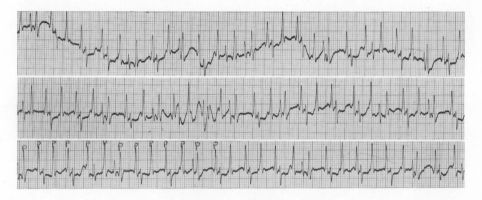

Fig. 12-9. Paroxysmal atrial tachycardia with block, recorded by an intracardiac electrode. In this very difficult rhythm, diagnosis was made by floating a recording wire into the right atrium. The tall complexes labeled *P* are the atrial complexes; when recorded from within the atria the P wave becomes a huge deflection, larger than the ventricular complex. The atrial rate is 188. Conduction to the ventricles varies, and precise diagnosis of this rhythm from the surface leads would have been almost impossible.

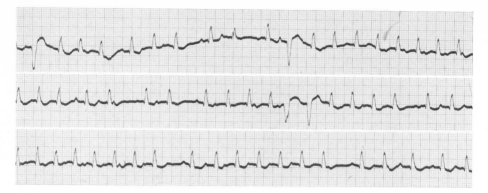

Fig. 12-10. Paroxysmal atrial tachycardia with A-V block interrupted by ventricular ectopic beats. The A-V block here is of the Wenckebach type. Note the midportion of the lower strip for the clearest evidence of the Wenckebach phenomenon. The ninth complex in this strip begins with a short P-R interval, which lengthens progressively until a P wave is blocked after the fifteenth ventricular complex. Again, ventricular ectopic firing is present, emphasizing the frequent association of these two manifestations of digitalis toxicity.

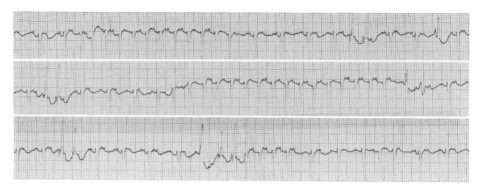

Fig. 12-11. Paroxysmal atrial tachycardia with A-V block. The interesting point about this specimen is the variation of conduction from 1:1 to 2:1 in various parts of the strip. In the upper left portion of the top strip a 2:1 ratio is present; this changes after the third ventricular beat to a 1:1 ratio, which continues for twelve beats, after which 2:1 conduction resumes. Aberrantly conducted beats are noted at various points throughout the tracing. A 1:1 conduction is unusual in paroxysmal atrial tachycardia with block but does occur, and it can be very confusing unless the possibility is kept in mind.

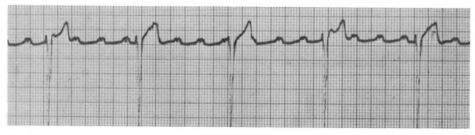

Fig. 12-12. Paroxysmal atrial tachycardia with complete A-V block. The atrial rate is 188; the ventricular rate is 46. The diagnosis of complete A-V block is established by the regular ventricular rhythm despite a changing relationship of atrial to ventricular complexes. It is clear that the atrial complexes have no connection with the slow ventricular rhythm.

NOTE: About one quarter of all cases of paroxysmal atrial tachycardia with A-V block are *not* produced by digitalis effect. When this arrhythmia appears in a patient who has *not* been taking digitalis and who does *not* have a low serum potassium, digitalis is often the best treatment.

Figs. 12-6 to 12-16 illustrate a number of types of paroxysmal atrial tachycardia with A-V block. The degree of A-V block may vary from first-degree to complete block. The paroxysmal atrial tachycardia may be a sustained rhythm or it may appear in short runs or bursts. Often the rhythm is so difficult to recognize on the electrocardiogram that only by application of vagal stimulation can the diagnosis be made. A large number of examples are presented here to emphasize the variety of forms the arrhythmia may assume and to help instill in the student a lively and continuing suspicion of this potentially lethal digitalis-induced arrhythmia.

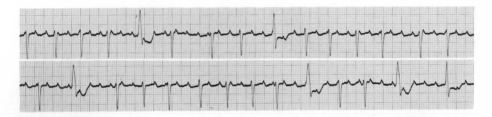

Fig. 12-13. Paroxysmal atrial tachycardia with block interrupted by frequent ventricular ectopic beats. Note fusion in the second ventricular premature beat in the top strip and in the last ventricular premature beat in the lower strip. Note erratically changing ratio of conduction to ventricles, producing a grossly irregular pulse, indistinguishable at the bedside from atrial fibrillation.

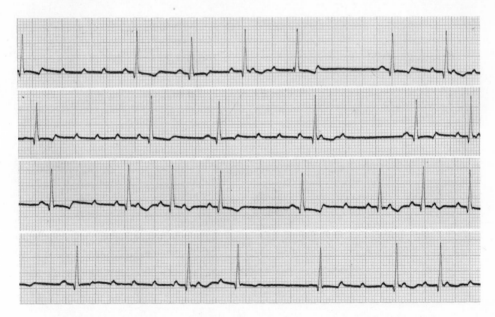

Fig. 12-14. Paroxysmal atrial tachycardia with block, occurring in short paroxysms.

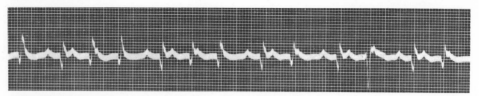

Fig. 12-15. Paroxysmal atrial tachycardia with A-V block of the Wenckebach type. Again, note complete irregularity of the ventricular rhythm.

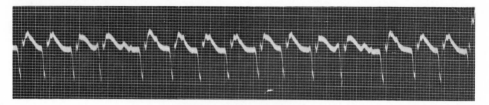

Fig. 12-16. Paroxysmal atrial tachycardia with Wenckebach type of A-V block. The P waves appear as notches on the T waves in most complexes. Helpful hint! Always look for the first beat after the pause to find P waves when they are difficult to see.

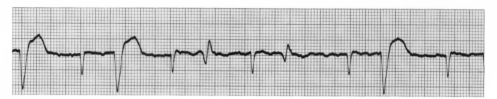

Fig. 12-17. Atrial fibrillation with ventricular ectopic beats forming a bigeminal rhythm.

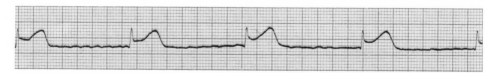

Fig. 12-18. Complete A-V block in the presence of atrial fibrillation.

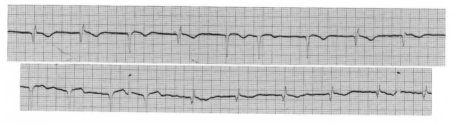

Fig. 12-19. Intermittent complete A-V block in the presence of atrial fibrillation. The first two complexes in the upper strip represent an ectopic rhythm arising in the A-V junction. The third, fifth, sixth, and seventh complexes in the top strip are irregularly spaced and are conducted down from the fibrillating atria. The last six complexes on the right-hand side of the bottom strip again represent the regular discharge of an ectopic pacemaker in the presence of atrial fibrillation.

Ectopic nodal and ventricular discharge interrupting atrial flutter and fibrillation

Most patients with atrial fibrillation or flutter receive digitalis; often, they receive too much. Many of these patients have been in congestive heart failure and have been given diuretic drugs without adequate potassium replacement. As a result, digitalis toxicity, enhanced by low serum potassium, is especially common in this group of patients. Be ready to *suspect* and to *detect* digitalis-toxic arrhythmias in the presence of atrial fibrillation or flutter.

Five types of mechanisms may operate:

1. Ventricular premature beats may interrupt atrial fibrillation or flutter (Fig. 12-17). These ectopic beats rarely present a diagnostic problem. Because of the very rapid atrial impulses, fusion beats are particularly common and help to establish the diagnosis of ventricular ectopic beating, as differentiated from aberrant conduction.

2. Complete A-V block may be induced by digitalis in the presence of atrial flutter or fibrillation. When this happens a regular, slow, ventricular rhythm will be detected, even though flutter or fibrillation are still present in the atria (Fig. 12-18). While this is a simple electrocardographic diagnosis, the clinical picture may confuse personnel in emergency rooms or coronary care units, with disastrous results.

The appearance of a regular, slow, ventricular rhythm in a patient with atrial flutter or fibrillation who has been receiving digitalis should be assumed to mean complete A-V block until an electrocardiogram can be recorded.

3. There may be a variable degree of A-V block with escape of a slow, ectopic rhythm for short periods (Fig. 12-19). In other words, there is complete failure of conduction through the A-V node for a period long enough to permit the escape of a lower ectopic pacemaker that sets a slow, regular, ventricular rhythm for a time until impulses from the atria again begin to reach the ventricles and dominate the rhythm.

Short intervals of slow, regular, ventricular rhythm interrupting atrial flutter or fibrillation indicate periods of complete A-V block. If the patient is taking digitalis, this is an indication to stop it.

4. An ectopic pacemaker may be accelerated to discharge in the normal range by the toxic effect of digitalis (accelerated idioventricular or idiojunctional rhythm). Some degree of A-V block delays conduction from the fibrillating atria enough to allow this accelerated ectopic rhythm to escape and set the rhythm of the ventricles, often for long periods. This kind of arrhythmia is an example of both types of toxic effect of digitalis—that is, vagal suppression of A-V conduction and acceleration of ectopic firing.

Appearance of a perfectly regular rhythm in the normal range interrupting atrial fibrillation in a patient taking digitalis does not necessarily mean that a normal sinus rhythm has been restored. It often means that an accelerated ectopic rhythm has appeared as a manifestation of digitalis toxicity. Again, digitalis should be stopped. (See Fig. 9-8.)

5. Junctional or ventricular paroxysmal tachycardia may appear in the presence of atrial fibrillation. The "ectopic accelerating" effect of digitalis may initiate paroxysmal tachycardia in the A-V junction or in the ventricles. This is of course the extreme manifestation of the ectopic accelerating effect of digitalis. A rapid, regular rhythm in the paroxysmal tachycardia range in a patient with atrial flutter or fibrillation who has been taking digitalis should again be regarded as evidence of a digitalis-toxic arrhythmia (Figs. 12-20 and 12-21). The drug should be stopped.

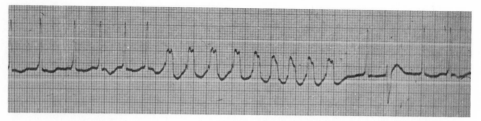

Fig. 12-20. Paroxysmal ventricular tachycardia interrupting atrial fibrillation.

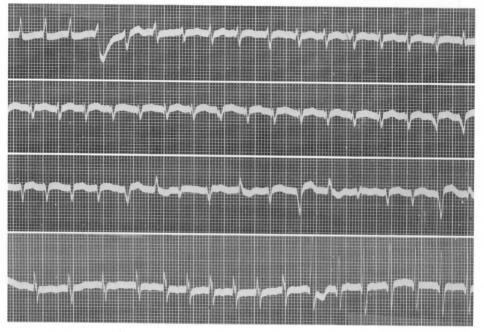

Fig. 12-21. Paroxysmal junctional tachycardia interrupting atrial fibrillation. Note characteristic A-V junctional tachycardia in the top two strips, termination of regular rhythm in the third strip, and, in the lowest strip, obvious atrial fibrillation.

In summary, regular ventricular beating in the presence of atrial arrhythmias, whether slow, normal, or rapid and whether present for prolonged periods or in short bursts, is very likely to represent digitalis toxicity, often of a dangerous degree. Always investigate this kind of arrhythmia carefully before making any further therapeutic decisions.

DIGITALIS DEPRESSION OF SINUS NODE FUNCTION

Toxic levels of digitalis may slow the S-A node because of excessive vagal effect. The most common result of this is sinus bradycardia.

More complex arrhythmias occur when the slow sinus rhythm permits the escape of ectopic rhythms arising in the A-V junction or in the ventricles (Fig. 12-22). The combination of sinus node slowing and idionodal or idioventricular accelerated escape

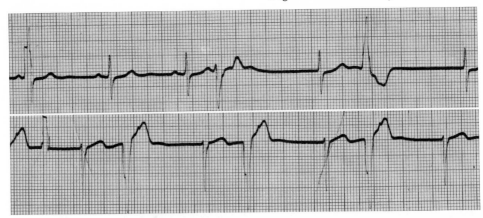

Fig. 12-22. Sinus bradycardia in the first three beats, ending with a ventricular ectopic beat. In the pause following this ectopic beat the junction escapes, setting a slow, regular junctional rhythm that is interrupted by ventricular ectopic beats forming a bigeminal rhythm.

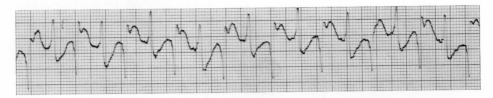

Fig. 12-23. Bidirectional ventricular tachycardia, a typically digitalis-toxic arrhythmia.

rhythms can produce bizarre and baffling arrhythmias. This type of arrhythmia should always alert the clinician to the possibility of digitalis toxicity.

The "sick sinus syndrome" is a term that describes a variety of malfunctions of the S-A node. Intermittent failure of the S-A node to discharge or to reach the atria is the common denominator (see Chapter 14). Whether the sick sinus syndrome can result from digitalis intoxication alone is not clear. It is certain, however, that a diseased S-A node that has been performing marginally can be transformed into a "sick sinus" by digitalis toxicity. The appearance of a sick sinus syndrome in a patient taking digitalis is a clear warning that digitalis toxicity may be present. If possible, the drug should be withdrawn.

BIDIRECTIONAL PAROXYSMAL VENTRICULAR TACHYCARDIA

This peculiar variety of ventricular tachycardia is usually a consequence of digitalis toxicity. The QRS complexes are wide, almost always with a right bundle branch block configuration; alternating complexes show a 180 degree change in direction, probably indicating alternating conduction down the two fascicles of the left bundle. The treatment is to stop digitalis (Fig. 12-23).

CLINICAL CONSIDERATIONS AND CORRELATIONS

This section starts with two commandments for any physician prescribing digitalis:

1. Never forget that digitalis is a toxic drug.
2. Never forget those clinical states that enhance toxicity of digitalis:
   a. Low serum potassium
   b. Chronic arterial hypoxemia
   c. Impaired renal function
   d. Old age

Low serum potassium

Diuretic therapy today is the most common cause of dangerous potassium loss. The thiazide drugs, furosemide, and ethacrynic acid are all drastic wasters of potassium. Any patient taking one of these drugs must be regarded as potassium-depleted within 3 or 4 weeks.

Loss of potassium from the gastrointestinal tract as a result of vomiting or during periods of nasogastric drainage may produce a dangerous drop in serum potassium levels.

Inadequate potassium replacement during periods of parenteral alimentation may also enhance digitalis toxicity. *Remember that a gradient exists between potassium levels within the cells and potassium levels in the serum; intracellular potassium may be dangerously depleted before the serum potassium begins to fall.*

Chronic arterial hypoxemia

Patients with any type of lung disease producing chronic arterial hypoxemia are extremely susceptible to the toxic effects of digitalis. In practical terms, this means that patients with chronic, obstructive lung disease or related syndromes must be digitalized with extreme caution, if digitalis is used at all. Animal experiments have demonstrated that arterial hypoxemia enhances the toxicity of digitalis two- or three-fold.

Impaired renal function

For years clinicians have known that older patients required less digitalis than younger ones, or, to state it another way, a dose of digitalis adequate for a patient of 40 is often toxic for a patient of 70. Marcus and associates have provided laboratory data to explain this phenomenon in the specific case of digoxin. They have shown that impaired renal function in older patients causes retention of the drug for long periods, with excessive accumulation from repeated daily doses.

Digitalis leaf contains some digoxin and is partly excreted through the kidneys; hence, renal function plays some role, although not a major one, in the toxicity associated with digitalis leaf.

Digitoxin is almost entirely excreted through the enterohepatic circulation into the gut; hence, it is not significantly affected by renal failure. *In any patient with impaired renal function and in any older patient who may have "subclinical" impairment of renal function, use very small doses of digoxin or digitalis leaf. Check BUN and creatinine in any older patient receiving digitalis.*

Total body mass helps determine digitalis requirements. Obviously, a 90-pound, elderly patient will require much less digitalis than a 200-pound, middle-aged individual; physicians are very likely to forget this. This may be another factor in the apparent increased sensitivity of aged patients to the toxic effects of digitalis.

TREATMENT

Prime treatment is to discontinue digitalis! It is possible to treat many cases of congestive heart failure without digitalis. Judicious combinations of diuretics, oxygen, xanthines, tourniquets, and other supportive measures can usually sustain the patient while digitalis levels fall from the toxic to the therapeutic range.

If a digitalis-toxic arrhythmia threatens life, specific therapy will be necessary. Paroxysmal tachycardia (particularly ventricular tachycardia), atrial tachycardia with A-V block, and any of the more severe forms of A-V block must be included in the category of life-threatening, digitalis-toxic arrhythmias. In a severely ill patient with borderline congestive failure, combinations of sinus node slowing with accelerated ectopic rhythms may cause a dangerous fall in cardiac output and will demand treatment.

Potassium

In any of the tachyarrhythmias resulting from potassium depletion and digitalis toxicity, administration of potassium is specific. If the patient's condition is not critical, give 40 mEq of potassium chloride orally initially and repeat the dose as indicated by the response of the arrhythmia. Frequent observation of the rhythm and serum potassium levels is necessary. Hourly doses may be necessary for a time, until some change in the rhythm can be observed or until serum potassium levels are noted to rise. In any critical condition, potassium should be given intravenously. From 60 to 80 mEq should be administered in 500 ml of normal saline. The anticipated period of administration should be about 4 hours, although this may vary a good deal. (The smaller doses of 20 mEq of potassium used in years past were probably inadequate, the potassium being "used up" during the infusion and the patient left no better off than before.) *Monitor the rhythm constantly while administering intravenous potassium and check serum potassium levels carefully.*

The total oral and intravenous doses of potassium cannot be precisely defined, since individual requirements will vary widely. There is no substitute for careful monitoring of the electrocardiogram and of the serum potassium levels in each patient receiving potassium.

This therapeutic use of potassium is for tachyarrhythmias. *When a normal sinus rhythm is associated with digitalis-induced A-V block, potassium should be given very cautiously and should never be administered intravenously, even when serum potassium levels are depressed.* In any patient with second- or third-degree A-V block, intravenous administration of potassium carries a real risk of cardiac arrest. If the potassium rises above a critical point, complete standstill may follow. In these patients, oral potassium only should be used. If the ventricular rate is dangerously slow, transvenous pacing should be used to maintain output while the digitalis effect abates.

Diphenylhydantoin

Diphenylhydantoin sodium (Dilantin), after many false starts as an antiarrhythmic agent, has emerged with one major, well-documented, specific use. Diphenylhydantoin is specific for digitalis-induced ventricular tachyarrhythmias, that is, paroxysmal ventricular tachycardia or repetitive ventricular firing induced by digitalis toxicity. The drug is *not* effective in ventricular tachyarrhythmias caused by myocardial ischemia, unlike lidocaine, quinidine, or procainamide.

Diphenylhydantoin has been reported to be beneficial in the treatment of atrial tachyarrhythmias, but in my experience this application of the drug has been disappointing.

Dosage. Diphenylhydantoin may be given orally or intravenously. In a classic study on the use of the drug, Bigger and associates defined the effective plasma level of diphenylhydantoin in the range between 10 and 18 μg/ml. These workers pointed out that a critical effective plasma level was essential before any antiarrhythmic activity of the drug could be demonstrated.

Intravenous administration. As recommended by Bigger, successive doses of 50 to 100 mg of diphenylhydantoin should be given every 5 minutes until the arrhythmia is abolished, until 1,000 mg has been given, or until undesirable effects appear. Intravenous diphenylhydantoin has been fatal. *Close electrocardiographic and clinical monitoring is essential.*

Oral administration. A loading dose would be 1,000 mg in divided doses on the first day, 500 to 600 mg on the second and third days, and subsequent maintenance doses of 400 to 500 mg per day.

WARNING: Even when diphenylhydantoin is given with these precautions it remains a dangerous drug. I know of two deaths following intravenous administration of diphenylhydantoin given with this exact protocol. The great majority of digitalis-induced arrhythmias will subside upon withdrawal of digitalis; *balance the risk of the treatment against the risk of the arrhythmia.*

Procainamide and lidocaine

These drugs may be used for digitalis-induced ventricular tachyarrhythmias. Doses and modes of administration are the same for any ventricular tachyarrhythmia. (See Chapter 19.)

Quinidine

In my opinion, this drug probably should never be used in digitalis-toxic arrhythmias; there may be the considerable danger of adding one toxic drug effect to another. Further, the less toxic modes of treatment already outlined will practically always end the arrhythmia.

Atropine

A-V block or S-A node depression may respond to atropine. When the ventricular rate is slowed significantly by either mechanism, intravenous atropine, 0.5 to 1.0 mg, should be tried. Opinions of the efficacy of the drug vary, but there is evidence that in acute overdosage, such as suicide attempts, atropine may be surprisingly effective. In chronic digitalis intoxication atropine is less helpful, but it should always be tried.

Pacing

If the ventricular rate has slowed critically as a result of A-V block or S-A node depression, ventricular pacing is essential. Maintenance of an adequate rate by pacing may prevent dangerous periods of ventricular asystole and will often be the key factor in sustaining cardiac output.

Isoproterenol

Do not use isoproterenol in the treatment of digitalis-induced A-V block; it may be very dangerous.

REFERENCES

Agarwal, B. L., and Agrawal, B. V.: Digitalis induced paroxysmal atrial tachycardia with AV block, Brit. Heart J. **34**:330-335, 1972.

Beller, G. A., and others: Digitalis intoxication: a prospective clinical study with serum level correlations, New Engl. J. Med. **284**:989-997, 1971.

Bigger, J., Jr., Schmidt, D., and Kutt, H.: Relationship between the plasma level of diphenyl-hydantoin sodium and its cardiac antiarrhythmic effects, Circulation **38**:363-374, 1968.

Ewy, G. A., and others: Digoxin metabolism in the elderly, Circulation **39**:449-453, 1969.

Harrison, D., Robinson, M., and Kleiger, R.: Role of hypoxia in digitalis toxicity, Am. J. Med. Sci. **256**:352-359, 1968.

Marcus, F. I., and others: The metabolic fate of tritiated digoxin in the dog: a comparison of digitalis administration with and without a "loading dose," J. Pharmacol. Exp. Ther. **156**:548-556, 1967.

13 Interference, dissociation, and confusion

Interference-dissociation, or A-V dissociation by interference, is a simple arrhythmia. The word "confusion" in the title of this chapter refers to the language often used to describe this arrhythmia.*

One should begin this chapter by learning four definitions.

Atrioventricular (A-V) dissociation. Sometimes the atria and the ventricles beat independently; when this happens, the atria are driven by an atrial pacemaker (usually the S-A node) and the ventricles by an ectopic pacemaker in the A-V junction or in the ventricles. The atrial and ventricular rhythms are thus separated from one another; they are independent, they are divorced. In the common term, they are "dissociated." *The term "atrioventricular dissociation," therefore, is a general term— it means simply that the atrial and ventricular rhythms are independent of one another.*

There are two causes of A-V dissociation:

1. Complete A-V block (Chapter 8)
2. Interference by an ectopic pacemaker

Interference. Every physician learns to use the word "interference" in premedical physics courses. It is used in hydraulics and optics. It describes what happens when two waves moving in opposite directions collide "head on" and are thus both extinguished (Fig. 13-1).

In electrocardiography the word "interference" means that an exciting wave that has started to progress across the heart meets an area of conducting tissue just discharged by another impulse and is therefore refractory. The original exciting wave is halted because of the "interference" of the second impulse (Fig. 13-2). A typical example of interference in the heart is the discharge of a pacemaker in the A-V junction just before the normal impulse from the S-A node reaches that area. The progress of the S-A wave through the A-V junction is halted, since the conducting tissues have just been discharged and are completely refractory. The ectopic focus has "interfered" with the passage of the S-A impulse from atria to ventricles.

When an ectopic pacemaker is discharging at about the same rate as the S-A node, each S-A impulse will encounter refractory tissue caused by the discharge of the ectopic pacemaker, and during this period no S-A impulses will reach the ventricles. There is, therefore, dissociation of atrial and ventricular rhythms caused by the inter-

---

*One learned investigator went so far as to propose the term "mutual extinction through refractoriness" as a substitute for the term "interference" as defined here!

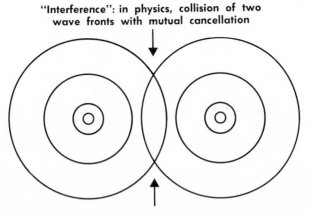

Fig. 13-1. "Interference" as defined in physics. The term implies the failure of an impulse to propagate in a particular direction because of "collision" with an opposite impulse.

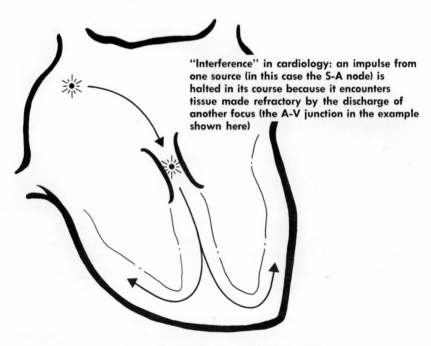

Fig. 13-2. "Interference" as defined in cardiology.

ference of an ectopic rhythm, or *interference-dissociation*. The term "atrioventricular dissociation by interference" is also used to describe this phenomenon. In simple terms, the ectopic beats "get in the way" of the S-A beats.

To avoid confusion, always use the word "interference" to refer to the effect of the ectopic pacemaker in halting the spread of the S-A impulse. The "lower" pacemaker (anatomically) is referred to as the interfering pacemaker. Thus a junctional pacemaker may interfere with the transit of the S-A impulses; a ventricular pace-maker might, at least in theory, prevent the spread of impulses from a junctional pacemaker.

Capture. It is almost impossible for two independent pacemakers to beat at the same rate for long periods of time. Sooner or later, they will get out of phase and a S-A impulse will reach the A-V junctional tissue between the discharges of the ectopic pacemaker. At this point, the A-V junctional tissue will be out of its re-fractory state and ready to conduct. The S-A impulse penetrates the A-V node and reaches the ventricles, producing a normal beat. This is called "capture" of the rhythm by the S-A node. The original word used for this by Mobitz was *verkettung* or *chaining*. The presence of capture beats is extremely important, as will be shown later in this chapter.

Complete atrioventricular (A-V) block. This term means specifically that the A-V conducting tissues are intrinsically incapable of conducting because of disease or intoxication; the tissues are functionally "dead."

With a clear understanding of the terms "A-V dissociation," "interference," "cap-ture," and "complete A-V block" the student should have few problems with the arrhythmias discussed in this chapter.

For practical, clinical purposes it is very important to distinguish between com-plete A-V block and interference-dissociation. The prognosis associated with ac-quired complete A-V block is always grave; the arrhythmia is often fatal. Inter-ference-dissociation, on the other hand, is usually a benign arrhythmia. Complete A-V block almost always requires permanent pacing. In many cases interference-dissociation requires no treatment at all. Thus, in both prognosis and in therapy, complete A-V block and interference-dissociation are two different entities—never confuse them! (Sometimes interference-dissociation and incomplete forms of A-V block may be combined, as illustrated in Chapter 15.)

MECHANISMS OF INTERFERENCE-DISSOCIATION

Figs. 13-3 to 13-6 illustrate four common mechanisms of interference-dissociation.

Accelerated A-V junctional or ventricular rhythm (Fig. 13-3). This is probably the most common cause of interference-dissociation. An ectopic pacemaker in the A-V junction or the ventricles begins discharging at a rate close to that of the S-A node, usually a little faster. As a result, the ectopic beats *interfere* with the transmis-sion of the S-A impulses to the ventricles, rendering the A-V conducting tissues re-fractory just before the arrival of the S-A impulse. As the reader already knows, these accelerated "idio-" rhythms are often produced by digitalis toxicity; interfer-ence-dissociation of this type, therefore, is frequently seen as a consequence of digitalis effect or digitalis toxicity.

Sinus bradycardia. A very slow sinus rate may permit an ectopic focus with a slightly more rapid inherent rate to begin discharging and take over the rhythm. In such cases, the basic cause of the interference-dissociation is simply the abnormally slow rate of S-A node discharge (Fig. 13-4).

Physiologic pause in the discharge of the S-A node. The pause after a premature beat or the slow phase of a sinus arrhythmia may allow an ectopic pacemaker to escape the influence of the S-A node and begin discharging. This is an example of the "escape" function of ectopic pacemakers, as illustrated in Chapter 4. The term "escape interference" is often used to describe this kind of interference-dissociation;

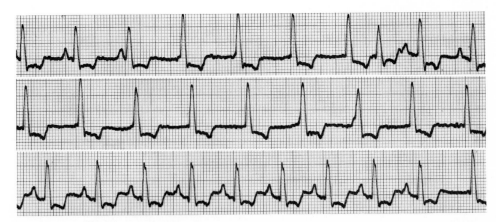

Fig. 13-3. Interference-dissociation. The cause of interference is an accelerated ectopic rhythm (probably junctional) discharging at a rate very close to the rate of the S-A node. In the top two strips the two rates are almost the same, producing "isorhythmic" dissociation in the first seven beats. Subsequently there are periods of sinus rhythm alternating with periods of accelerated junctional rhythm. In the bottom strip, sinus rhythm is present throughout until the last beat, when a pause in S-A node firing allows the junctional pacemaker to escape in the last visible beat.

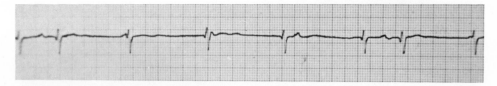

Fig. 13-4. Interference-dissociation caused by an escape junctional rhythm in the presence of sinus bradycardia. The dominant rhythm is A-V junctional; the second and seventh ventricular complexes represent capture beats. Note the slow sinus rate that permits the escape of the ectopic pacemaker. The first visible P wave is conducted to the ventricles, producing the second ventricular complex; the second P wave is partially "buried" in the third ventricular complex; the third P wave is "buried" in the fourth ventricular complex; the fifth P wave comes too soon after a junctional beat to be conducted to the ventricles; and the sixth captures a beat.

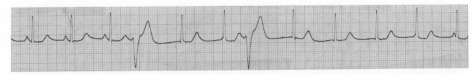

Fig. 13-5. Escape of A-V junctional rhythm in the pauses following premature ventricular beats. Normal sinus rhythm is present in the first three beats; a PVC follows. In the postectopic pause the junctional pacemaker, which has a rate very close to the S-A rate, "escapes" and sets the rhythm, with the exception of one PVC, for the rest of this strip. Notice the reappearance of a sinus P wave in the last two beats of the strip, just ahead of the ventricular complexes. Unless there is interruption by another PVC, the rapid S-A rate will ultimately capture the rhythm.

it is a useful term, since it indicates that the basic cause of the arrhythmia is failure of the S-A node rather than acceleration of an ectopic pacemaker (Fig. 13-5).

Paroxysmal tachycardia. This is a special type of interference-dissociation. Paroxysmal tachycardia arising in the A-V junction or in the ventricles often suppresses the S-A node by retrograde conduction across the atria. Occasionally, when there is no such retrograde conduction, the atria may beat independently under the control of the S-A node. A type of interference-dissociation results. If the rate of paroxysmal tachycardia is not too rapid, occasional S-A beats will be conducted to the ventricles, interrupting the paroxysmal tachycardia (Fig. 13-6).

CAPTURE BEATS

Capture beats refer to S-A beats that reach the A-V conducting tissues *between* ectopic beats, find these tissues ready to conduct, and reach the ventricles. In colloquial terms, a S-A impulse will "sneak through" between ectopic beats to reach the ventricles and produce a normal S-A beat (Fig. 13-7, *A*).

It is very important to look for capture beats. They give the clinician his only chance to see whether the A-V conducting tissues are capable of functioning or not. In other words, the differential diagnosis between interference-dissociation and complete A-V block rests on the detection of capture beats. If an occasional S-A impulse

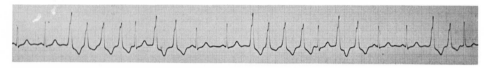

Fig. 13-6. Paroxysmal ventricular tachycardia with occasional captures by the S-A node. Notice normal QRS's interrupting runs of ventricular tachycardia: this means that the atria are beating independently during the ventricular tachycardia; atrial impulses occasionally reach the ventricles. Independent atrial rhythm during parosyxmal tachycardia is one special form of "interference-dissociation."

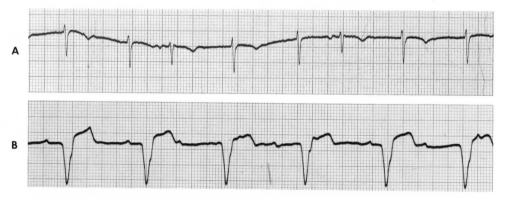

Fig. 13-7. A, Interference-dissociation with capture. The third and sixth beats are capture beats, interrupting an A-V junctional rhythm. **B,** Failure of capture. In this strip the atrial rhythm is rapid and slightly irregular, possibly a result of a chaotic atrial rhythm. The ventricles are responding to an idioventricular pacemaker with a relatively slow regular rhythm. Note that in no case do P waves reach the ventricles to produce a "capture" beat. The conclusion, therefore, is that the A-V conducting tissues are intrinsically unable to conduct and that A-V block is present.

does reach the ventricles with a normal P-R interval, it is conclusive evidence that the A-V dissociation is caused by the interference of an ectopic pacemaker and not by complete failure of function of the A-V conducting tissues.

On the other hand, if an S-A impulse arrives at the A-V conducting tissues when these tissues are free of the influence of the ectopic pacemaker, and if this S-A impulse does not capture the ventricular rhythm, the conclusion is that the A-V conducting tissues are intrinsically incapable of functioning and that complete A-V block does exist (Fig. 13-7, *B*).

A prolonged P-R interval in a capture beat is evidence of a diseased but still functioning set of A-V conducting tissues, corresponding to incomplete forms of A-V block.

To summarize, in the course of interference-dissociation an S-A impulse will eventually reach the A-V conducting tissues at a time when transmission to the ventricles is possible, as far as the effect of the ectopic pacemaker is concerned. If transmission does not take place at such a time—if no capture beats result—then true A-V block must be present.

The practical, clinical importance of this distinction can hardly be overemphasized.

ISORHYTHMIC DISSOCIATION

Sometimes the S-A node and the interfering ectopic focus discharge at exactly the same rate for a time. The P waves and the QRS complexes will be exactly superimposed, not because they have any relation but by simple coincidence of rate. This isorhythmic firing never continues indefinitely. Sooner or later, the two pacemakers get "out of phase" and a S-A impulse slips past the ectopic pacemaker to capture a beat (Fig. 13-8).

CLINICAL SIGNIFICANCE AND TREATMENT

To understand the clinical significance and treatment of interference-dissociation, simply refer to the four basic causes of the arrhythmia.

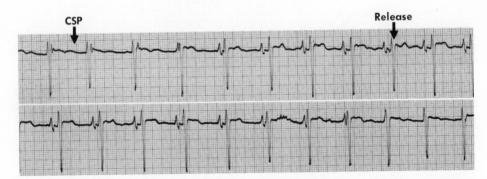

Fig. 13-8. Isorhythmic dissociation. In the left-hand portion of the upper strip a junctional rhythm is present. Note P waves "hidden" in the ventricular complexes, indicating isorhythmic beating. With carotid sinus pressure the A-V junctional rhythm is slowed relatively more than the S-A rhythm, and the sinus P waves are conducted to the ventricles for a short time. In the right-hand side of the bottom strip there is slight acceleration of the junctional pacemaker, which "takes over" the rhythm, again becoming isorhythmic—meaning that the sinus P waves and the junctional ectopic beats occur at almost exactly the same time.

Accelerated A-V junctional and ventricular rhythms. (See Chapter 5.) These accelerated "idio-" rhythms are often associated with digitalis toxicity, which is why the statement is often made that "interference-dissociation is frequently a manifestation of digitalis overdosage."

Slowing of S-A node. If the cause of the interference-dissociation is an escape phenomenon associated with a very slow S-A node discharge, acceleration of the S-A rate by atropine or acceleration of the atrial rate by atrial pacing may be required as a temporary measure.

Physiologic pauses. If postectopic beat pauses are responsible for releasing an ectopic pacemaker, which then sets up an interference-dissociation pattern, it sometimes may be necessary to suppress the ectopic focus, thus doing away with the pauses that are the causes of the arrhythmia in the first place. (Note again Fig. 13-5.)

Paroxysmal tachycardia. Here, the treatment and the prognosis, of course, depend on the type of paroxysmal tachycardia present. Whether there is a dissociated atria or retrograde conduction from the paroxysmal tachycardia across the atria is an interesting phenomenon of no real significance. The paroxysmal tachycardia is the arrhythmia to be treated.

In any patient with compromised cardiac function the appearance of an A-V junctional or ventricular rhythm may drop the cardiac output critically, thus endangering life. Idionodal and idioventricular rhythms, whether normal or accelerated, are not to be regarded lightly in such patients. One should try to suppress such rhythms by speeding the S-A node with atropine or by atrial pacing. The 25% increase in cardiac output associated with a resumption of normal sinus rhythm may well be lifesaving.

REFERENCES

Ballarino, M., Rumolo, R., and Folli, G.: La dissociazione per interferenza in corso di blocco atrioventricolare, Cuore Circ. **43**:291-314, 1959.

Marriott, H. J. L., Schubart, A. F., and Bradley, S. M.: A-V dissociation: a reappraisal, Am. J. Cardiol. **2**:586-605, 1958.

Miller, R., and Sharrett, R.: Interference dissociation, Circulation **16**:803-829, 1957.

Mobitz, W.: Zur Frage die atrioventrikulären Automatie: die Interferenz dissoziation, Duetsch. Arch. Klin. Med. **141**:257, 1923.

Phibbs, B.: Interference, dissociation, and semantics: a plea for rational nomenclature, Am. Heart J. **65**:283-285, 1963.

14 Sick sinus syndrome

Sick sinus syndrome is a wastebasket diagnosis; it happens to be a very useful wastebasket, which includes a group of related arrhythmias with one feature in common, *subnormal function of the S-A node.*

In the first edition of this text I stated: "Sinoatrial block is a minor arrhythmia of no clinical significance." This statement was absolutely wrong—the only consolation is that this was an opinion held almost universally at that time. In fact, the sick sinus group of arrhythmias *is* clinically significant; it produces major symptoms, and it is associated with a surprising morbidity and a certain mortality.

A sick sinus appears in one of three different forms:

1. *Persistent sinus bradycardia.* The S-A node takes an abnormally long time to build up its charge to a firing level; as a result, the S-A rate is very slow. This will appear clinically as persistent sinus bradycardia.

2. *Sinoatrial (S-A) block.* This means that an area of "exit block" exists in the tissue immediately around the S-A node. Even though the S-A impulses build up normally, they do not reach the atrial tissue because they cannot traverse the area of refractory tissue that surrounds the S-A node. Clinically, this will appear as a sudden pause in the rhythm of the heart. On the electrocardiogram there will be simply a short period when there are no P waves.

3. *Sinus bradycardia or S-A block interrupted by periods of rapid, supraventricular arrhythmias* (paroxysms of atrial fibrillation, flutter, paroxysmal atrial or junctional tachycardia, or multifocal atrial tachycardia). The exact cause of this kind of inadequate S-A function is not clear. Recent pathologic studies suggest strongly that degeneration of the cells of the S-A node is almost always involved. Frequently, there is massive replacement of the pacemaking cells by scar tissue. Coronary artery disease and other forms of degenerative disease of the myocardium are the common causes of this syndrome.

CLINICAL MANIFESTATIONS

The symptoms of the sick sinus syndrome are clear-cut and easy to relate to the arrhythmia. They are:

1. Vertigo or syncope associated with the slow S-A discharge or with the pauses in S-A discharge
2. During periods of supraventricular tachyarrhythmia, sensations of "fluttering in the chest," "pounding of the heart," or any of the other symptoms associated with any tachyarrhythmia

135

Death from sick sinus syndrome per se seems rare, but arterial embolism is surprisingly common, specifically in the bradycardia-tachycardia form of the arrhythmia.

The symptoms of syncope, vertigo, and discomfort associated with tachyarrhythmias are often so severe that the patient is substantially incapacitated.

Disease of the A-V conducting tissues is commonly associated with the sick sinus syndrome. Whenever a patient presents with evidence of a sick sinus, a careful search for evidence of A-V block of any degree should be included in the diagnostic studies.

TYPES OF SICK SINUS SYNDROME

Sinus bradycardia. Sinus bradycardia is an obvious form of the syndrome and needs little comment. The patient with an excessively slow sinus rate that does not respond appropriately to exercise is probably suffering from sick sinus syndrome. Further studies should be carried out to verify the diagnosis (see below).

Prolonged postectopic pauses (Fig. 14-1). When a premature beat discharges the S-A node, the pause following such a beat should not be longer than the normal P-P interval when the S-A node is discharging normally. Thus the time interval from a premature atrial beat to the next normal sinus beat should not be longer than the interval between two sinus beats. This is also true when a junctional or ventricular ectopic beat fires retrogradely across the atria, with the same effect of discharging the sinus node prematurely.

If the sinus node is "sick" it will take longer than normal to rebuild the charge to a firing level, and the postectopic pause will be prolonged. The two ectopic atrial beats at the beginning of Fig. 14-1 are followed by a very long pause (over 2 seconds, counting from the second ectopic P wave). During this time no sinus P wave appears, and the pause is ended only by an ectopic beat arising in the A-V junction. In the right-hand side of the strip the P-P interval between two normal sinus beats is noted to be about 1 second. Hence, the diagnosis of sick sinus syndrome is substantially established by the prolonged pause following the ectopic atrial firing. This is a very common phenomenon, and the physician should be alert for its appearance, since it is highly suggestive of a serious sick sinus syndrome.

Sinoatrial block. Figs. 14-2 and 14-3 illustrate the phenomenon of S-A block. In the top strip of Fig. 14-2, the sinus is discharging normally at a rate of about 74. After the fourth beat there is a sudden pause when no P waves appear for almost 1½ seconds (1,400 msec). At the right-hand end of the strip the sinus rhythm is interrupted by a premature junctional beat, which is followed by a sinus P wave. The sinus P wave is not conducted to the ventricles, since the A-V conducting tissues have been rendered refractory by the premature beat. There is a long pause following this P wave, during which no P wave appears (over 1 second), ending with another junctional ectopic beat, this time appearing as an escape ectopic beat. In the bottom

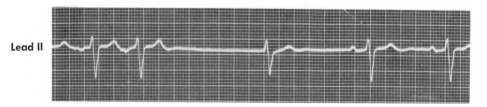

Fig. 14-1. Sick sinus syndrome with prolonged postectopic pause (see text).

strip, on the left-hand side, a nonconducted sinus P wave is followed at a normal P-P interval by a run of sinus beats. After the eighth beat on the bottom strip, there is another pause during which no P wave appears (1,200 msec), after which the sinus node resumes firing at the same rate as before the pause.

Thus there are three episodes of S-A node block when an inexplicable pause in the discharge of the S-A node appears abruptly without any preceding disorder of rhythm (see top left, top right, and bottom right of this strip). This is evidence of a sick sinus syndrome of the S-A exit block type.

Fig. 14-3 is a second example of S-A block. Here the pause between the second and third beats on the strip is exactly double the interval between the first two beats. This is the classic type of S-A block when 2:1 block appears. In other words, one

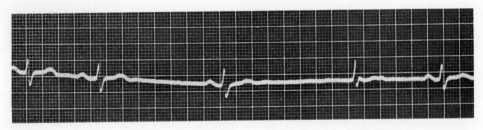

Fig. 14-2. Sick sinus syndrome; S-A block (see text).

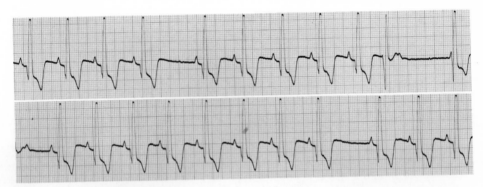

Fig. 14-3. Sick sinus syndrome; S-A block. Note junctional escape following pause (see text).

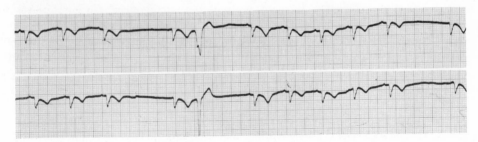

Fig. 14-4. Sick sinus; S-A block with 9:5 ratio of conduction from S-A node to atria (see text).

S-A impulse is blocked before it reaches the atria, while the following S-A impulse is conducted normally across the atrial tissues. Exit block around the S-A node will sometimes present an exact 2:1 or 3:2 ratio, but more often it will be an irregular phenomenon, as in Fig. 14-2, with prolonged pauses in the discharge of the S-A node.

Fig. 14-4 illustrates severe S-A block with very prolonged pauses terminated by ectopic beats. On the right-hand side of both strips there are five sinus beats before the pause. This pattern was repeated over and over for long periods in this patient. The P-P interval during regular beating is 800 msec. The interval between the last sinus beat and the first beat after the pause is 3,200 msec. This cycle is repeated precisely. It is thus clear that after five conducted beats, three beats are blocked. It is also clear that the S-A node goes on building up and discharging at exactly the same rate; the arrhythmia results from the fact that the S-A impulse does not reach the atria because of recurrent exit block—five beats are conducted, while the succeeding three are not. The total pattern could be described as an 8:5 S-A block.

Bradycardia-tachycardia syndromes. Fig. 14-5 illustrates one type of the bradycardia-tachycardia syndrome. Here a slow sinus rate with frequent pauses is interrupted by a paroxysm of atrial flutter. The long pause following the fourth beat in the top strip ends with an A-V junctional escape beat, which is followed by a paroxysm of atrial flutter. After the end of the atrial flutter, there are rare P waves in the right-hand side of the bottom strip and there are a number of A-V junctional escape beats. This patient described distressing "pounding and beating of the heart" together with episodes of syncope. The combination of symptoms made it necessary for him to leave his job as a bus driver.

Fig. 14-6 illustrates another type of bradycardia-tachycardia syndrome. At the left-hand side of both strips a sinus bradycardia is apparent (rate about 53). Note that the sinus P wave recorded in the V_1 position is chiefly negative. An ectopic atrial beat, wide and notched, appears after the second beat in both strips. This is followed by a run of junctional beats with what seem to be retrograde P waves. In the upper strip, after a short pause the junctional rhythm resumes, again with varying retrograde conduction. One sinus beat follows the first run of junctional rhythm, and, after a premature ventricular beat, another series of junctional beats is noted. The same sequence of events is apparent in the bottom strip. Here the tachycardia phase of the bradycardia-tachycardia syndrome consists of multiple junctional beats that appear rapidly and irregularly. In addition, frequent premature ventricular contractions (PVC's) are noted, which is a very unusual finding in bradycardia-tachycardia syndrome. This patient described distressing vertigo and near-syncope that appeared erratically without any reference to obvious inciting factors.

Fig. 14-7 illustrates many of the features of the bradycardia-tachycardia type of sick sinus syndrome. In many parts of the tracing there are no P waves for long periods and junctional ectopic beats are noted. Where P waves are present, the P-R interval is greatly prolonged, indicating disease of the A-V conducting tissues. In the top, second, fifth, and bottom strips there are short runs of atrial tachyarrhythmia, probably a coarse atrial fibrillation or possibly an atrial flutter, for 1 or 1½ seconds. This combination of an atrial tachyarrhythmia, with long sinus pauses that allow a slow, junctional pacemaker to set the rhythm, with A-V block is a severe form of the sick sinus bradycardia-tachycardia syndrome. This patient suffered from repeated episodes of syncope and had had one transient episode of hemiplegia, which in the light of current knowledge probably represented an arterial embolus.

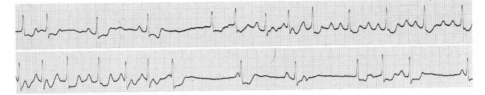

Fig. 14-5. Bradycardia-tachycardia type of sick sinus (see text).

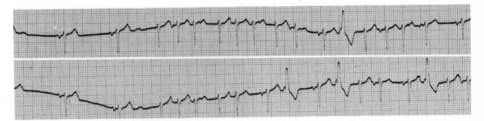

Fig. 14-6. Bradycardia-tachycardia type of sick sinus (see text).

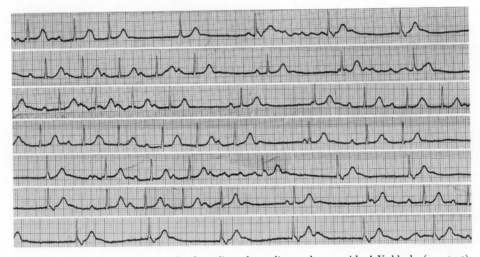

Fig. 14-7. Sick sinus combining bradycardia-tachycardia syndrome with A-V block (see text).

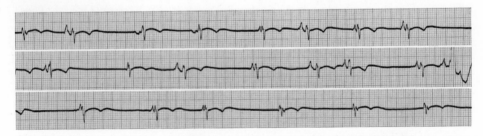

Fig. 14-8. Sick sinus syndrome manifested after cardioversion of atrial fibrillation (see text). (Courtesy Dr. George A. Spikes, Douglas, Ariz.)

Fig. 14-8 represents a common manifestation of sick sinus syndrome—that is, sub-normal S-A node function in the period immediately following electroversion for atrial fibrillation. This is the type of arrhythmia that Lown first described as a "sick sinus." P waves are few and appear at irregular intervals. There are many junctional beats, and there are some inverted P waves that may represent retrograde conduction from the nodal ectopic focus. The appearance of this kind of sick sinus following electro-version probably means that the patient will not be able to maintain a normal sinus rhythm. It implies severe disease of the S-A node, and it is safe to assume that this kind of patient will revert to fibrillation in a relatively short time.

STEPS IN DIAGNOSIS OF SICK SINUS SYNDROME

When a patient describes episodes of syncope or severe vertigo, always consider the sick sinus syndrome as a differential diagnosis. When any of the obvious electro-cardiographic manifestations of the sick sinus syndrome illustrated here are present, the diagnosis has substantially been established.

When the diagnosis is not clear-cut from a resting electrocardiogram, it is well to have a Holter type of monitor recording done for 12 or 24 hours. Often the ar-rhythmia will be manifest and can be correlated with the patient's symptoms. Un-fortunately, this apparatus is not always available, and, in my view, the fees charged by many cardiologists and internists for recording and interpreting such tracings are excessive. Much of the time, therefore, the clinician will be well advised to try some simpler and less expensive steps in diagnosis.

Atropine administration. Intravenous atropine (approximately 1 mg) is useful in the detection of a sick sinus. The normal response to intravenous atropine is an in-crease in the pulse rate by a factor of 50% to 60%. A sick sinus node will respond sluggishly or occasionally will not respond at all. A rate increase of 25% or less has been described as characteristic of the sick sinus syndrome.

Overdrive suppression of S-A node. Almost every hospital with a coronary care unit owns a pacer of some variety. It is a simple matter to thread a pacing catheter into the right atrium and institute rapid atrial pacing. One characteristic of the sick sinus already pointed out is a slow recovery time following a premature discharge. This effect is greatly accentuated following a period of rapid atrial pacing. The aver-age clinical pacing unit has a maximum rate of about 150 beats, which is adequate for this purpose. If the atrium is paced at a rate of 150 for 30 seconds or more and the pacer is then turned off, the time required for recovery may give the key to the diagnosis. With a healthy S-A node, the recovery time—the time from the end of pacing to the first normal sinus beat—will be about 1½ seconds. In the presence of a sick sinus, the pause will be 3 or more seconds. While introducing a pacing catheter to the right atrium may seem an impressive procedure to most clinicians, it is really simpler and safer than electroversion of any arrhythmia and it represents utilization of equipment and skills that should be available to any physician caring for cardiac patients.

Carotid sinus stimulation. Carotid sinus stimulation may be hazardous in patients with a severe sick sinus syndrome and probably should be carried out only with careful monitoring and with the possibility of atrial pacing if prolonged asystole results. A minority of patients with the sick sinus syndrome show excessive carotid sinus sensitivity and will manifest long pauses following stimulation of the carotid sinus. This is probably the least useful of the diagnostic modes listed here in defining the syndrome.

Holter monitor recording. Continuous Holter monitor recording, when available and when not prohibitively expensive, is extremely useful and may be the definitive mode of diagnosis.

TREATMENT

Treatment of the sick sinus syndrome has been discouraging. Drugs such as atropine or isoproterenol have little long-term effect in speeding the rate of discharge of the S-A node. While the various tachyarrhythmias suggest the need for suppressive drugs, the possibility that these drugs may dangerously depress an already subnormal S-A node makes their use hazardous.

When the patient's symptoms are severe enough to justify intervention, ventricular pacing probably gives the best long-term results. It may be difficult for many clinicians to accept the idea of a drastic intervention, such as implantation of a pacemaker, for what was formerly thought to be a minor arrhythmia. Keep in mind, however, that this arrhythmia is often disabling and is attended by significant morbidity. A great many of the more severe types of the sick sinus syndrome certainly warrant implantation of a pacemaker.

The bradycardia-tachycardia types of sick sinus are probably helped by the use of suppressive drugs *after* a ventricular pacemaker has been inserted. The choice of drug will vary with the type of tachyarrhythmia present, but digitalis is probably the preferred agent in the great majority of patients. Before instituting antiarrhythmic therapy, however, it is well to await the patient's response to pacing, since in many cases this seems to do away with the need for any other therapy.

SUMMARY

Always suspect the sick sinus syndrome when vertigo or syncope appear without some obvious cause. Investigate for evidence of sinus bradycardia, S-A block, or the bradycardia-tachycardia syndrome using the diagnostic modes outlined. If there is a question, do not hesitate to call for the services of a skilled cardiologist who can use overdrive pacing and timed ectopic beat stimulation to help with the diagnosis. When the syndrome produces disabling symptoms, and particularly when the syndrome is of the bradycardia-tachycardia type, proceed with definitive therapy, ventricular pacing, and possible subsequent use of antiarrhythmic drugs.

REFERENCES

Davies, M., and Pomerance, A.: Quantitative study of ageing changes in the human sinoatrial node and internodal tracts, Brit. Heart J. **34**:150-152, 1972.

Ferrer, M.: The sick sinus syndrome in atrial disease, J.A.M.A. **206**:645-646, 1968.

Mandel, W., and others: Evaluation of sino-atrial node function in man by overdrive suppression, Circulation **44**:59-66, 1971.

Narula, O., Samet, P., and Javier, R.: Significance of the sinus-node recovery time, Circulation **45**:140-158, 1972.

Rubenstein, J., and others: Clinical spectrum of the sick sinus syndrome, Circulation **46**:5-13, 1972.

15 Some complex arrhythmias

This chapter presents a group of complex disorders of rhythm, all relatively common and all clinically significant, that involve specific prognostic and therapeutic decisions.

INTERFERENCE-DISSOCIATION COMBINED WITH A-V BLOCK

In the tracing in Fig. 15-1 a slow regular rhythm is noted, interrupted by occasional premature beats. The basic rhythm consists of regular, narrow QRS complexes that are not preceded by P waves. The diagnosis is therefore an idiojunctional rhythm. Sinus P waves are visible randomly scattered throughout the tracing; hence, one may conclude that this is a true interference-dissociation pattern, with the atria being driven by the S-A node and the ventricles by a junctional pacemaker. The first P wave in the top strip is conducted to the ventricles. This is the explanation of the premature beats noted here, at the right-hand end of the top strip, in the fifth beat of the second strip, and in the fourth beat of the bottom strip. In other words, occasional capture of the ventricular rhythm by the sinus node does take place.

Upon examination of the P-R interval of these capture beats, it is clear that the A-V node is diseased, since the P-R interval is approximately .28 second in each conducted sinus beat. The sinus rate is very slow (about 33). The final diagnosis of this arrhythmia, therefore, is (1) severe sinus bradycardia, probably sick sinus syndrome, (2) interference-dissociation with slow A-V junctional rhythm, and (3) incomplete A-V block. (The exact degree of block cannot be determined, since only occasional P waves are conducted to the ventricles. If every P wave were conducted, it might be possible to decide whether 2:1 block, Wenckebach phenomenon, or the like would result. All that can be said at this time is that the A-V conducting system is diseased but is still capable of functioning.)

HIGH DEGREE OF A-V BLOCK WITH INTERFERING A-V JUNCTIONAL RHYTHM

The tracings in Fig. 15-2 were recorded on a 56-year-old woman during the course of viral myocarditis. The tracings were recorded on a three-channel electrocardiograph. Inspection of Fig. 15-2, *A*, reveals P waves at a regular, moderately rapid rate (125). Sinus tachycardia is therefore present. A much slower ventricular rhythm is noted, with a rate of about 45. It is clear that some type of A-V block is present; the question is: "Is the block complete or not?"

Careful inspection of the first four complexes on this strip reveals a curious rela-

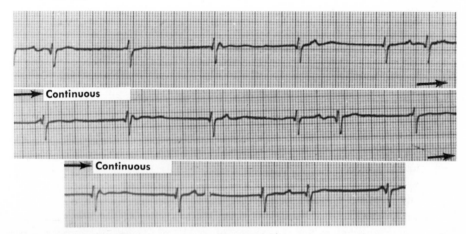

Fig. 15-1. Interference-dissociation with A-V block. (See text.)

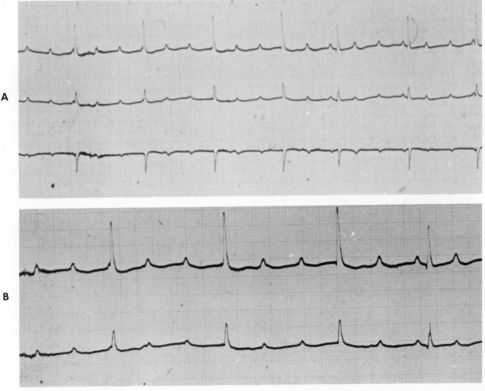

Fig. 15-2. A and **B,** Interference-dissociation with A-V block. (See text.)

tion; every third P wave seems to occur just before or during a ventricular complex, while the other two P waves in each cycle are clearly blocked. The ventricular rhythm is regular for the first four beats, and at this point one would strongly suspect complete A-V block. However, the fifth ventricular complex is premature; this complex is preceded by a P wave at a normal conducting distance, .16 second. The appearance of premature ventricular beats interrupting a basically regular ventricular rhythm practically always rules out complete A-V block.

When a premature beat is preceded at a normal conducting distance by a P wave, the possibility of capture of the ventricular rhythm by the sinus node is very strong. In this rhythm the fifth beat actually represents a normal sinus beat, while the other ventricular complexes are clearly produced by an ectopic pacemaker arising in the A-V junction. It is curious that the junctional pacemaker happens to have a rate that is almost exactly one third the rate of the S-A node, so that the junctional QRS complex coincides almost precisely with every third sinus P wave. The presence of the capture beat tells the physician that the A-V conducting tissues are capable of functioning.

There is also clearly some degree of block, since many P waves are not conducted, but the essential point here, as demonstrated by the capture beat, is that the block is not complete. It is clear that the block would be of high degree, that is, 3:1 or 4:1. It is impossible to tell the degree of block, since the junctional pacemaker "gets in the way" of the third P wave and there is no chance for propagation to the ventricles because of the interference of the ectopic pacemaker.

Diagnosis of this complex rhythm, therefore, is a high degree of A-V block, not complete, combined with an interfering A-V junctional rhythm.

Fig. 15-2, *B*, shows the same phenomenon greatly magnified. Notice the slightly different QRS configuration of the capture beat (the last beat) compared to the beats arising in the junctional pacemaker. As the reader already knows, differences in morphology between QRS complexes produced by a normally conducted beat and those arising in the A-V junction are common. The crucial point, of course, is that the ectopic QRS complexes are narrow, indicating that they do not arise in the ventricles.

ACCELERATED ECTOPIC RHYTHM WITH A-V BLOCK

Fig. 15-3 illustrates an arrhythmia seen very commonly with acute rheumatic carditis. This was noted in a 16-year-old boy with fulminating acute rheumatic fever with carditis. P waves are noted at regular intervals, with a rate of about 74; hence, the S-A node is discharging normally. A rapid, regular ventricular rhythm is noted with a rate of approximately 88. There does not seem to be any connection between

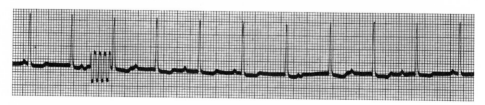

Fig. 15-3. Interference-dissociation and A-V block with acute rheumatic carditis. (See text.)

the P waves and the ventricular complexes. The conclusion, therefore, is that an accelerated junctional rhythm is producing the ventricular rate, while the S-A impulses never reach the ventricles. The question here is: "Are the A-V conducting tissues viable or not?"

To answer this, note the P waves following the fourth, eighth, and ninth ventricular complexes. These P waves should capture the ventricular rhythm and produce a premature beat, out of phase with the regular rhythm of the A-V junctional pacemaker. One can state that these P waves should capture the ventricular rhythm because the time interval between these P waves and the preceding QRS complexes is sufficiently long to have permitted the A-V conducting tissues to recover from the A-V junctional beat and to be ready for transmission of the S-A impulses to the ventricles. The fact that no such transmission occurs indicates that the A-V conducting tissues are not capable of normal function; some degree of block must exist in the A-V conducting system. The exact degree of block cannot be determined because the rapid firing of the ectopic pacemaker in the A-V junction never allows a pattern of block to be observed. This combination of A-V block and accelerated junctional rhythms in acute rheumatic carditis is practically always transitory; reversion to normal sinus rhythm is the rule.

CONCEALED CONDUCTION INTO A-V NODE

This common phenomenon is illustrated in Fig. 15-4. A normal sinus rhythm is present, interrupted by a premature atrial beat (the second complex). Between the fifth and sixth sinus beats there is a ventricular ectopic beat. This beat is *interpolated*, that is, there is no compensatory pause after the ectopic beat. The P-R interval of the first sinus impulse following the ventricular premature contraction is much longer than in all the other sinus beats (.18 versus .14 second). The explanation for this is that the ectopic impulse that arose in the ventricles penetrated the A-V node

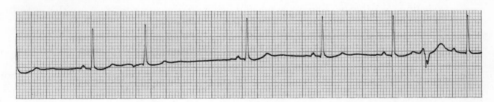

Fig. 15-4. Concealed conduction from ventricular ectopic beat into A-V node. (See text.)

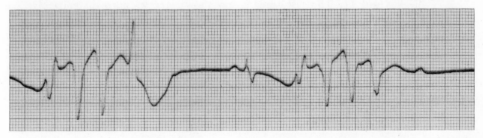

Fig. 15-5. Concealed conduction from runs of ventricular tachycardia, producing A-V block. (See text.)

from below, partially exhausting the structure. The next sinus P wave found some part of the A-V conducting tissues (probably the A-V node) still in a relative refractory state, and the impulse was conducted more slowly than normal.

Prolongation of the P-R interval in the first sinus beat following an interpolated ventricular ectopic beat is the most common manifestation of concealed conduction into the A-V node. Remember that passage of the activating wave through the A-V node and bundle of His does not produce a deflection on the surface electrocardiogram; hence, conduction into these structures can often be detected only by inference, that is, by the behavior of the next sinus beat passing through the A-V conducting tissues.

Fig. 15-5 shows another example of concealed conduction, with grave consequences. On the left-hand side of the strip there are four ventricular ectopic beats forming a run of paroxysmal ventricular tachycardia. Note that these beats arise in more than one focus. In the center of the strip a sinus beat is noted with a P-R interval of .20 second. Following this is another run of ventricular tachycardia, after which another P wave is noted. This P wave is *not* followed by a ventricular response. Since the first sinus beat on the strip is conducted normally to the ventricles and since there is no transmission from atria to ventricles between the first and second visible P waves, why is the second P wave not conducted to the ventricles?

During the period of ventricular tachycardia there has been some retrograde conduction into the A-V conducting tissues, which has exhausted some part of the A-V system so that at the time of the second visible P wave, the A-V conducting system is completely refractory. This is an example of ventricular firing with concealed conduction that produces a significant degree of A-V block.

One would also conclude that there was disease of the A-V conducting tissues of some degree, since healthy A-V conducting tissues would have recovered from the concealed conduction of the ventricular tachycardia by the time of arrival of the second visible P wave.

The point to be made here is that concealed conduction may play a role in aggravating A-V block, and in some clinical situations eradication of the source of the concealed conduction may ameliorate the degree of block.

RATE-DEPENDENT BUNDLE BRANCH BLOCK

Block in any of the conducting tissues of the heart may be rate-dependent. Diseased conducting tissues may be capable of conducting at a slow rate but may manifest delayed conduction or may fail to conduct at all at a higher rate. A common example of this is rate-dependent bundle branch block. Fig. 15-6 is a good illustration of this phenomenon. The first four beats on this strip show typical left bundle branch block (lead I). The last three beats show *narrow,* normal ventricular complexes. Careful examination of the rate shows that during the period of left bundle branch

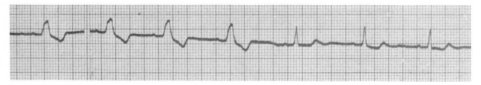

Fig. 15-6. Rate-dependent bundle branch block. (See text.)

block the rate is 68; during the period of normal intraventricular conduction the rate is 64. This slight difference in rate is enough to allow the left bundle branch to recover from its refractory period and conduct normally.

Fig. 15-7 shows just how confusing this kind of rate-dependent change may be. The top strip shows a typical bundle branch block pattern with a ventricular ectopic beat (the second beat) and a fusion beat (the fourth beat). In the bottom strip the fourth ventricular complex is narrow. There is a long pause in the ventricular rhythm before the normally conducted beat that explains the difference; the bundle branch block is *rate-dependent,* and a sufficient pause in the ventricular rhythm allows the diseased bundle to recover and conduct normally for one beat. Note the premature atrial

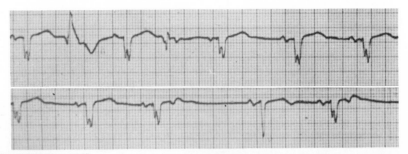

Fig. 15-7. Rate-dependent bundle branch block. (See text.)

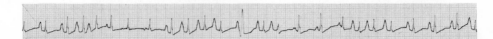

Fig. 15-8. Chaotic atrial rhythm. Note erratic variation in contour and timing of P waves (patient with severe, chronic, obstructive pulmonary disease).

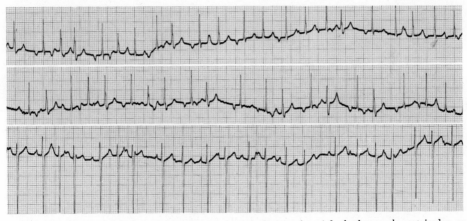

Fig. 15-9. Chaotic atrial rhythm. Note gross irregularity of atrial rhythm and ventricular response, together with extreme variation in contour of P waves (chronic, obstructive lung disease with digitalis intoxication).

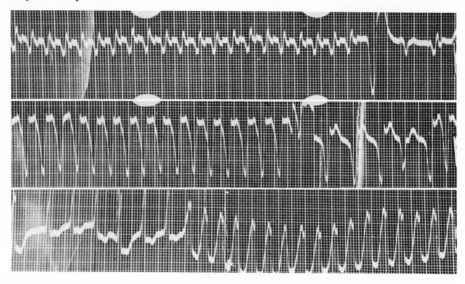

Fig. 15-10. Chaotic ventricular rhythm. Terminal rhythm with paroxysms of ventricular tachycardia from several foci.

beats following the third and fifth ventricular complexes in the bottom strip; these atrial impulses are blocked, hence the pause in the ventricular rhythm.

Always keep in mind the possibility of rate-dependency when considering bundle branch block. When one is differentiating between bundle branch block and ventricular ectopic firing, this phenomenon can sometimes be very confusing.

CHAOTIC RHYTHMS

The adjective "chaotic" simply means multifocal ectopic firing. Figs. 15-8 and 15-9 illustrate chaotic atrial rhythm. Note the multiple ectopic P waves with varying contours and different rates of coupling that form a grossly irregular rhythm. Chaotic atrial rhythm is seen very commonly in association with chronic, obstructive lung disease. Arterial hypoxemia seems to play a major role in producing the arrhythmia. Digitalis toxicity may also contribute. Chaotic atrial rhythm in combination with chronic, obstructive lung disease carries a grave prognosis; some workers have postulated a mortality of as high as 60% within 6 months of the appearance of this arrhythmia.

Fig. 15-10 is an example of chaotic ventricular rhythm. Chaotic ventricular rhythm could also be termed "multifocal ventricular tachycardia." The prognosis is always extremely grave, and in the great majority of cases the arrhythmia progresses to ventricular fibrillation. Prompt, drastic intervention is required with antiarrhythmic drugs and possibly with electroversion.

REFERENCES

Chung, E.: Appraisal of multifocal atrial tachycardia, Brit. Heart J. **33**:500-504, 1971.
Fletcher, E., and others: Atrioventricular dissociation with accrochage, Brit. Heart J. **33**:572-577, 1971.
Friedberg, H., and Schamroth, L.: Concealed Wenckebach phenomena in the left bundle-branch, Brit. Heart J. **34**:370-373, 1972.

Massumi, R., Amsterdam, E., and Mason, D.: Phenomenon of supernormality in the human heart, Circulation **46**:264-275, 1972.

Moe, G., and Mendez, C.: Functional block in the intraventricular conduction system, Circulation **43**:949-954, 1971.

Paulay, K., Damato, A., and Bobb, G.: Atrioventricular interaction in isorhythmic dissociation, Am. Heart J. **82**:647-653, 1971.

16 Fatal arrhythmias; arrhythmias in the coronary care unit

The two fatal arrhythmias are ventricular fibrillation and ventricular standstill. These are combined in the chapter on arrhythmias in the coronary care unit for a very good reason—before the development of coronary care units, successful treatment of either of these arrhythmias was very rare.

VENTRICULAR FIBRILLATION

Ventricular fibrillation is a feeble, rapid, twitching motion of the ventricles (Fig. 16-1). Since the ventricles have stopped beating and have begun twitching, no blood is being pumped; the patient loses consciousness at once, and unless resuscitation begins, he will be dead in 10 minutes or less. The mechanism of ventricular fibrillation was unlocked by the discovery of the "vulnerable zone" of the heart by Lown and his group. Briefly, during a short period (.04 second) just before the peak of the T wave, the heart is "vulnerable." If an appropriate stimulus is applied to the heart during this period, ventricular fibrillation will follow. *For clinical purposes, it is important to remember that a ventricular ectopic beat often serves as the stimulus that produces ventricular fibrillation when such a beat occurs in the vulnerable zone of the T wave* (Fig. 16-2).

Evidence of irritability in ventricular foci is often a warning that ventricular fibrillation impends. Some simple criteria for "ventricular ectopic irritability" are:
1. Presence of frequent ventricular ectopic beats (six or more a minute)
2. Presence of multifocal ventricular ectopic beats
3. Runs of ventricular ectopic beats forming short bursts of ventricular tachycardia
4. Ventricular beats occurring in the vulnerable zone of the T wave

The presence of any of these types of ventricular ectopic firing in a patient suffering from any kind of myocardial ischemic process is a signal to begin prompt suppressive therapy with lidocaine, procainamide, or quinidine.

VENTRICULAR FLUTTER

Ventricular flutter is an often misunderstood "first cousin" of ventricular fibrillation. Ventricular flutter describes a rapid, feeble contraction of the ventricles, strong enough to be felt when the heart is held in the hand and powerful enough to generate an electrocardiographic signal, but not adequate to pump any significant amount of blood (Fig. 16-3). The electrocardiographic distinction between ven-

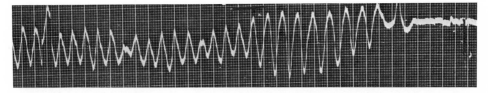

Fig. 16-1. Ventricular fibrillation with spontaneous end of the arrhythmia and resumption of normal beating.

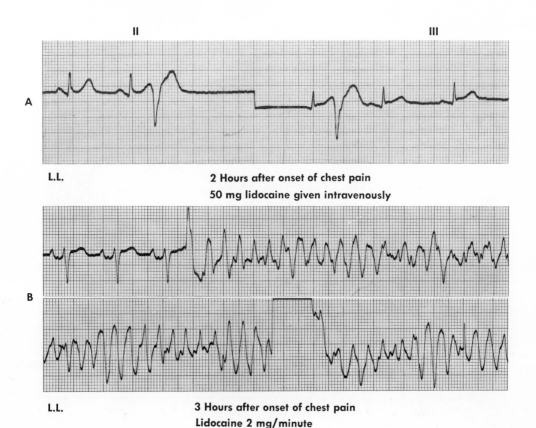

Fig. 16-2. A, PVC's occurring in or close to the vulnerable zone of the T wave. **B,** PVC occurring in the same patient in the vulnerable zone of the T wave, triggering an episode of ventricular fibrillation. (Courtesy Dr. Gorden Ewy.)

tricular flutter and ventricular tachycardia is important. In ventricular tachycardia there are clear-cut ventricular complexes and it is possible to distinguish between the QRS and the T waves. In ventricular flutter all morphology is lost and there are simple, large "saw teeth" with no apparent distinction between QRS or T waves. With the appearance of ventricular flutter the patient usually loses consciousness; it is practically always followed by ventricular fibrillation in a short period. *Ventricular flutter is an indication for defibrillation, just as much as ventricular fibrillation, since it is a fatal arrhythmia.*

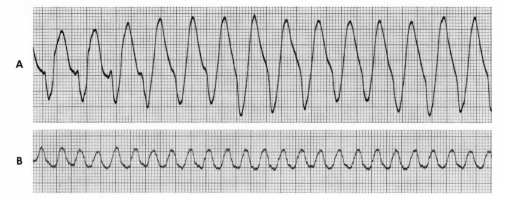

Fig. 16-3. A, Ventricular flutter following ventricular tachycardia. **B,** Ventricular flutter. Note characteristic rapid rhythm with absence of any definition of QRS or T components of the ventricular complex.

VENTRICULAR STANDSTILL

Complete asystole, or ventricular standstill, may be the result of two different processes.

First, progressive A-V block may result in long periods of asystole. (Presumably, the junctional and ventricular ectopic pacemakers have been overwhelmed by some pathologic process and are not capable of generating an escape rhythm.) Second, complete hypoxic arrest of the heart rhythm may take place, with progressive loss of pacemaker function in the atria, in the A-V junction, and, finally, in the ventricles. Such "hypoxic standstill" usually ends with a very slow idioventricular rhythm, with wide, irregularly spaced, ventricular complexes.

TREATMENT

A tidal wave of literature about cardiac resuscitation has engulfed the medical public in recent years. I will not attempt to duplicate the basic instructions about cardiac defibrillation and resuscitation, which are familiar to practically everyone, including first-aid workers. Instead, I will attempt to point out some common errors and reasons for failure in cardiac resuscitation.

Ventricular fibrillation

The best treatment is prevention! Be alert for the signs of ventricular ectopic firing and treat them aggressively.

Defibrillation. Medical science does progress. Studies in progress by my colleague, Dr. Gordon A. Ewy, indicate that commercial defibrillators usually do not perform as claimed by the manufacturers; further, they reveal certain hazards hitherto unsuspected. Read Chapter 21 carefully. The data on defibrillation and cardioversion given there represent new knowledge that should be familiar to every physician who performs defibrillation or cardioversion.

Drugs. Suppressive drugs are of little use in the treatment of ventricular fibrillation. Lidocaine, procainamide, and quinidine are relatively ineffectual. Epinephrine, on the other hand, when injected into the ventricle or intravenously, has been shown to increase the likelihood of successful defibrillation, probably because of better "tone" of the myocardium. Inject 0.1 ml of 1:1,000 solution directly into the ventricle through the chest wall. REMEMBER: The heart is not beating—injecting drugs into the motionless heart is an exercise in futility. The drug will not leave the chamber unless cardiac massage is continued.

The only other drug useful in ventricular fibrillation is sodium bicarbonate, which should be administered in any cardiac arrest. One ampule (44.6 mEq) should be administered every 3 minutes until the heart is beating and the patient is adequately ventilated.

Ventricular standstill

Pacing. Ventricular pacing is of course the ideal treatment for ventricular standstill. This means that a pacer has to be introduced percutaneously through a median basilic, subclavian, or jugular vein. I believe that subclavian puncture is dangerously overused by physicians who were trained in this technique as residents and who have become enthralled by their own dexterity in this simple maneuver. Subclavian vein puncture is dangerous; it often produces pneumothorax and sometimes causes death when the subclavian artery is torn. It is just as simple—and perfectly safe—to insert a catheter into a median basilic vein and thread it into the right ventricle with electrocardiographic or fluoroscopic monitoring. (See Chapter 20.) The unfortunate tendency of physicians to use new and intriguing invasive techniques, with little regard for mortality or morbidity, promotes many needless disasters. The popularity of the "subclavian stick" is a case in point.

If a patient goes into ventricular standstill as a result of progressive A-V block, the standstill should have been anticipated and a pacer should be in position, with function tested, before asystole appears.

When asystole appears suddenly, the catheter must be threaded into the right ventricle while massage and artificial respiration are being administered. This is considerably more difficult, but it can be done.

Drugs. Two drugs are useful in the treatment of cardiac arrest: epinephrine and calcium chloride.

One milliliter of a 1:1,000 solution of epinephrine should be injected into the ventricle repeatedly every few minutes until there is a response. If epinephrine alone is not effective, 2.5 ml of a 10% solution of calcium chloride is injected and may be repeated in 3 or 4 minutes.

REMEMBER: *There is no point in injecting a drug into the heart unless continuous massage is carried on to expel the drug into the coronary circulation.*

The prognosis of standstill depends on the source or type of standstill. When progressive A-V block results in periods of asystole, there is a reasonable hope that pacing may sustain an adequate cardiac rate with ultimate recovery. When total hypoxic depression of the ventricular conducting system produces standstill, chances of recovery are very small. I have seen one patient with this type of standstill who did recover, however; a conscientious physician will always use every possible means of resuscitation.

Open chest massage. In the wave of enthusiasm that followed the discovery of closed chest massage, the medical world seemed to forget two important facts about open chest or direct massage of the heart.

1. Direct massage of the heart is much more effective, in terms of cardiac out-

put, than closed chest massage. Cardiac output with open chest techniques may double the maximum that can be achieved by closed chest massage.

2. Frequently, direct massage of the heart will start a heartbeat when all other methods fail.

Open chest massage, of course, involves a thoracotomy and a considerable morbidity; it is to be recommended only under certain, limited circumstances, but in those circumstances it will occasionally save lives.

Before giving a patient up for dead, open chest massage of the heart should be considered first:

1. *If* the resuscitation is taking place in a well-equipped emergency room, coronary care unit, or operating room
2. *If* the patient is of an age and state of health that make resuscitation seem a reasonable possibility
3. *If* all other methods have failed and the operator is ready to give up

Thus, before admitting that the 36-year-old father of a family could not be resuscitated and was in effect dead when the ventricles were still fibrillating, open chest massage should be tried. I have personally resuscitated two patients by open chest massage when all other modes failed. Each time, the only regret was that open chest massage had not been used earlier, since some cerebral damage attended the prolonged use of closed chest methods.

TECHNIQUE. To open a chest for cardiac massage, make a quick incision from a few centimeters left of the left sternal margin to the anterior axillary line in the fourth or fifth interspace. Incise rapidly but not too deeply; it is very easy to nick an enlarged ventricle. The second cut should take the operator through the intercostal muscles. The operator now slides the right hand sideways between the ribs, twisting the hand and spreading the ribs apart, so that the palm of the hand faces upward. The hand is thrust into the chest cavity so that the fingers and palm are dorsal to the heart *and the thumb rests outside the chest on the sternum.* (This precaution is very important, since a thumb applied to a ventricle during massage often produces massive myocardial necrosis.) Massage is then effected by bringing the fingers and palm up against the sternum, compressing the ventricles. *It is especially important to release quickly to produce a brisk diastolic filling between squeezes.* The effectiveness of open chest massage in producing bounding arterial pulses is astonishing.

If a prolonged period of massage seems necessary, the ribs are incised and rib spreaders are inserted. In most cases, however, by simply forcing the ribs apart with the hand and using this simple method of massage, very efficient expulsion of blood from the heart can be obtained for an adequate period.

Open chest massage is also helpful in allowing the physician to gauge the state of the ventricular musculature. If the heart continues to lie flabbily in the hand with no evidence of contractility after administration of epinephrine and calcium and after adequate massage, it is not likely that further attempts to resuscitate will help. On the other hand, if the heart muscle begins to manifest tone and if the physician is aware of a firm, hard, "squeezing" character of the heartbeat, he can assume that there is indeed a significant amount of viable myocardium with which to work.

Again, open chest massage is to be used as a last resort in certain selected cases in appropriate areas. Within these restrictions, however, the method can certainly save lives.

ARRHYTHMIAS IN THE CORONARY CARE UNIT

First, an editorial comment! *The essential element in any coronary care unit is a well-trained nurse looking at a large oscilloscope pattern of an electrocardiogram.* An appalling quantity of expensive electronic gimmickry has been unloaded on a gullible medical public—the yield can be described charitably as minimal. Alarm systems practically never function properly; they are triggered by artifacts so often that nurses in coronary care units almost always turn them off. Memory loops may be of some value. Histograms and other paraphernalia, while possibly helpful in amassing statistics for research, are of no appreciable immediate benefit to patients. The moral of this is that the physician who is organizing a coronary care unit in a clinically oriented hospital should think in terms of well-trained coronary care nurses, large oscilloscopes with multiple-sweep speeds and lead selection capability, and a switching system that permits activation of a central electrocardiographic write-out from each bedside in the unit. Beyond these basic components, other equipment at this date has proved to be largely window dressing.

Some rules for evaluation of arrhythmias following myocardial infarction or acute myocardial ischemia should be observed.

Any paroxysmal tachycardia complicating myocardial infarction should be ended promptly. The fall in output and the excessive demand for myocardial oxygen will certainly jeopardize the patient's life.

Atrial flutter or fibrillation complicating myocardial infarction or ischemia always should be ended promptly. The rapid ventricular rate and the drop in cardiac output associated with lack of atrial synchronization may precipitate shock or congestive failure, with lethal results.

A-V junctional or ventricular rhythms ("idio" rhythms), whether slow or in the accelerated range, should be watched very carefully. Such idiojunctional or idionodal rhythms are often described as benign arrhythmias, but this is not always true. Again, the fall in cardiac output that follows absence of atrial synchronization may not be tolerated in a patient who has suffered a severe myocardial infarction. If the blood pressure falls during one of these rhythms or if the patient shows other signs of circulatory embarrassment, it is well to attempt treatment. Treatment, of course, will depend on the reason for the escape of the ectopic pacemaker. Generally speaking, two types of treatment are used:

1. Increase the S-A rate by intravenous injection of 0.5 to 1 mg of atropine. This will frequently accelerate the S-A node so that the ectopic pacemaker is depressed and the hemodynamic effects of a normal synchronized heart are realized.

2. If atropine does not accomplish this result, atrial pacing is often needed. Properly carried out, this is a completely safe, quick procedure that will often increase cardiac output critically. The "atrial kick" effect may be the only resource left to a patient with a severely damaged myocardium. When shock or failure are serious problems, this resource should never be overlooked.

Severe sinus bradycardia, as in a sick sinus syndrome, without an ectopic escape rhythm, may also depress cardiac output in a critically ill patient. Again, atropine or atrial pacing should be utilized to generate maximum cardiac performance. There are some very simple rules about the relation of A-V block to myocardial infarction.

1. A-V block accompanying infarction of the anterior wall is a very grave

arrhythmia. This type of block usually implies disease of the left anterior descending branch of the left coronary artery, and the site of the block is usually in the upper parts of both bundle branches rather than in the A-V node. A patient with an anterior myocardial infarction with severe first-degree block or any of the higher types of A-V block (second- or third-degree) faces a mortality of 75% to 85%. It is very likely that this patient will progress to complete standstill. *Always* insert a transvenous pacing catheter into the right ventricle when a patient with an anterior myocardial infarction manifests second- or third-degree A-V block. When first-degree A-V block presents with severe P-R prolongation, it is probably wise to insert a catheter prophylactically. A depressing fact is that even these precautions will not increase survival much, but it is well to do whatever can be done. The pacing may be useful in sustaining cardiac output, which is almost certainly going to be compromised in this type of infarction.

2. A-V block associated with inferior wall or posterior wall infarction is not as severe as A-V block associated with anterior myocardial infarction. First-degree block with inferior or posterior wall infarction does not call for intervention. Many competent observers feel that second-degree block with these types of infarction does not call for intervention unless the ventricular rate is slowed critically.

I have seen patients progress to asystole punctuated by ventricular fibrillation when A-V block is complicated an inferior wall infarction. Since the introduction of a pacing catheter is a simple and substantially harmless affair, I feel that in any second-degree block, and certainly in all cases of third-degree block accompanying an inferior or posterior wall infarction, a pacing catheter should be inserted and tested for capture.

ADDENDUM

I include some notes on cardiac resuscitation, or things that are usually forgotten in the hurry and confusion of a cardiac arrest!

1. Always begin resuscitation with a couple of thumps with the closed fist on the sternum. Surprisingly often, this will start a heartbeat.

2. The angel of death always hovers near the scene of a cardiac arrest—often the dread messenger is disguised as a physician, bearing in his incompetent hands the equipment for endotracheal intubation. If anyone except an expert anesthesiologist or otolaryngologist approaches the patient with equipment for endotracheal intubation, send him off on some other errand or else use forcible restraint! The mortality from cardiac arrest is high enough without compounding it by incompetent attempts at intubation of the trachea. If proper mouth-to-mouth resuscitation or bag resuscitation is being carried on and if the patient is not obstructed by saliva or vomitus, there is no immediate reason to intubate.

I have watched many physicians without special training waste 30 to 60 seconds in futile attempts to intubate the trachea. During this time the heart was not being massaged and no artificial respiration was being administered. The patient's brain was becoming hypoxic and the level of carbon dioxide in the blood was mounting logarithmically. *Every 30 seconds without massage or respiration tips the scales heavily against the patient's survival.*

Two good working rules governing endotracheal intubation during cardiac arrest are:

a. Nobody except those skilled in endotracheal intubation and ready to accomplish this in 10 or 15 seconds should ever try to intubate a patient during cardiac arrest.

b. No matter who attempts the intubation, somebody should count seconds during the intubation attempt. After 10 seconds, the attempt should be halted while the heart is massaged and artificial respiration is continued for another 20 or 30 seconds. Certainly, no more than 15 seconds should be allowed to pass without cardiac massage and artificial respiration. I have sometimes found it necessary to remove the intubator and his equipment from the patient's proximity forcibly while restoring massage and respiration. When a patient's life is at stake, the most extreme measures are justified!

3. Observe the phenomenon of the uselessly employed physician. When a patient has suffered a cardiac arrest and the nursing personnel are massaging the heart and ventilating the lungs by mouth-to-mouth or bag-assisted breathing, it is the height of folly for a physician to bustle up to the bedside and take over the job of cardiac massage. The prime function of a physician should be to get a needle or preferably a plastic cannula into a vein so that intravenous medication can be administered promptly. He may also be helpful in interpreting the rhythm on the oscilloscope. The physician should be firmly directed toward these two fields of possible usefulness. A cutdown set should be made available, and if the veins are not easily punctured, he should be encouraged to make an entry into the venous system by incision as promptly as possible. The enthusiast who insists on subclavian puncture at this point should also be removed from the scene of action. A pneumothorax would probably put the patient past any hope of resuscitation. Since all that is needed is a line into the venous system for administration of medication, subclavian cannulation at this time is absolutely unjustified. It imposes one more hazard on a patient already in desperate straits.

REFERENCES

Bloomfield, S., and others: Quinidine for prophylaxis of arrhythmias in acute myocardial infarction, New Engl. J. Med. **285**:979, 1971.

DeSanctis, R., Block, P., and Hutter, A., Jr.: Tachyarrhythmias in myocardial infarction, Circulation **45**:681-702, 1972.

Ewy, G. A.: Ventricular arrhythmias following acute myocardial infarction, Southwestern Med. **52**:75-85, 1971.

Rokseth, R., and Hatle, L.: Sinus arrest in acute myocardial infarction, Brit. Heart J. **33**:639-642, 1971.

Rotman, M., Wagner, G., and Wallace, A.: Bradyarrhythmias in acute myocardial infarction, Circulation **45**:703-722, 1972.

17 Wandering pacemaker; pre-excitation; criteria of aberration; parasystole

WANDERING PACEMAKER

This simple arrhythmia may be a source of much confusion. It is a harmless variant of the sinus rhythm. As a rule, a sinus rhythm is characterized by P waves with identical shapes that indicate that the pacemaker arises in exactly the same position and follows exactly the same course across the atria with each beat. In the condition called wandering pacemaker, the shape of the P wave changes progressively; for instance, it may progress from upright to flat, to inverted, back to flat, and then back to upright (Fig. 17-1). Presumably the site of the pacemaker is "wandering" around the S-A node, and possibly even back and forth in the area between the S-A and A-V nodes. A wandering pacemaker should not be confused with ectopic atrial firing. Note that none of the atrial complexes is premature; note further that the variation in P-P interval is about that to be expected with a sinus arrhythmia. Wandering pacemaker is a common finding of no significance. Never confuse it with ectopic firing.

IDIOATRIAL RHYTHM

In contrast to the common wandering pacemaker, it is possible to see a true "idio" rhythm arising in an ectopic atrial focus (Fig. 17-2). In the top strip the first seven beats are normal sinus beats with a rather small P wave. The eighth beat begins a series of complexes that are almost identical in spacing but that manifest one important difference—the P waves abruptly change their shape and size. In the right-hand side of the strip the P waves are large and spiked; these obviously arise from a different focus in the atrium. The same kind of change is noted (in a different lead) in the lower strip.

Idioatrial rhythm probably has no particular significance and falls within the class of "harmless variations of rhythm."

PRE-EXCITATION (WOLFF-PARKINSON-WHITE SYNDROME)

Some patients have a congenital "short-cut" or bypass between the atria and ventricles that seems to "short circuit" the normal A-V nodal pathway. A-V conduction is rapid; as a result, the P-R interval is short. The exciting wave enters the ventricles by a slightly aberrant course, which results in a QRS that is abnormal in shape. The specific abnormality associated with pre-excitation is noted in the first

158

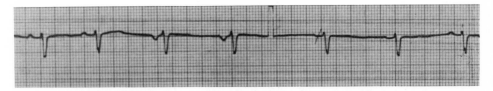

Fig. 17-1. Wandering pacemaker. Note alteration in P wave configuration from upright to deeply inverted, to isoelectric, and then back to upright.

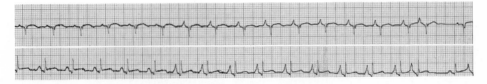

Fig. 17-2. Idioatrial rhythm. (See text.)

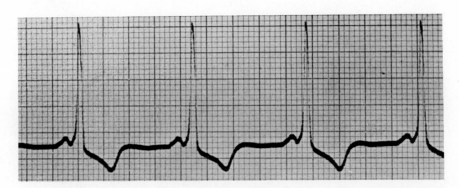

Fig. 17-3. Pre-excitation (Wolff-Parkinson-White syndrome), Type A, lead V_1.

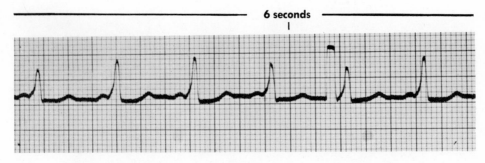

Fig. 17-4. Pre-excitation, Type A, lead V_1. Note the very wide delta-R wave.

.02 or .03 second of the ventricular complex and consists of a small, slurred portion of the R wave referred to as the "delta-R" wave.

Pre-excitation falls into one of two general patterns—Type A or Type B. Type A is characterized by a ventricular complex in lead V_1 that consists of an R wave with a typical delta-R (Figs. 17-3 and 17-4). (Remember that in Type A pre-excitation the QRS complex in V_1 resembles A.) Type B pre-excitation is characterized by delta-R and R waves in lead V_6, while V_1 has a normal configuration, that is, it consists of a small R with a deep S (Fig. 17-5).

The pre-excitation in Type A probably lies in the lateral basal portion of the septum so that the aberrant fibers "short circuit" into the left bundle branch system. In Type B pre-excitation the anomalous conducting pathway lies to the right, connecting the right atrium and the right ventricle; the exciting impulse "short circuits" into the right bundle branch system.

The diagnosis of pre-excitation therefore rests on:
1. A short P-R interval (.10 second or less)
2. Widening of QRS complexes (.11 second or longer)
3. An interval from the beginning of P to the end of the ventricular complex that is the same as the interval in normal sinus beats

In other words, the widening of the QRS compensates for the shortening of the P-R.

The Lown-Ganong-Levine syndrome is a variation of the Wolff-Parkinson-White syndrome, except that the QRS complex in the former is normal in shape and is narrow (.08 second wide).

Patients with pre-excitation of any type are susceptible to episodes of paroxysmal tachycardia, which are sometimes incapacitating and may call for drastic measures. If there is a single specific indication for the use of beta-adrenergic blocking agents

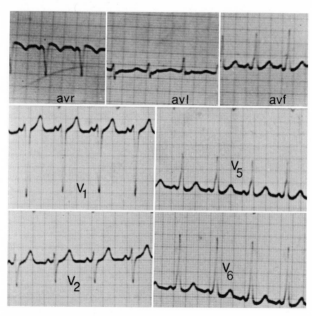

Fig. 17-5. Pre-excitation, Type B. Note normal configuration of right precordial leads with delta-R wave over left precordium.

in treating arrhythmias, it is probably in the treatment of the supraventricular tachycardias associated with pre-excitation. In this class of arrhythmia such agents are uniquely useful. In extreme cases surgical division of the anomalous pathway has been attempted, but the results have not been satisfactory.

ABERRANT INTRAVENTRICULAR CONDUCTION VERSUS VENTRICULAR ECTOPIC FIRING (ASHMAN PHENOMENON AND MARRIOTT'S CRITERIA)

As noted in Chapter 6, it is often difficult and sometimes impossible to decide whether a wide ventricular complex is the result of aberrant intraventricular conduction or of ventricular ectopic firing. Several rules may help in making this distinction, although they are not infallible.

Ashman phenomenon

The Ashman phenomenon is basic to an understanding of aberrancy. Briefly, this phenomenon is based on a simple fact of physiology; the slower the heart rate, the longer the refractory period, both absolute and relative (effective and functional). Thus, at a slow rate (50 to 60), there will be a very long period following each beat when a subsequent beat will not be conducted at all or will be conducted aberrantly (Fig. 17-6). As the heart rate speeds, the refractory period shortens. To state it differently, the longer the R-R interval, the longer the refractory period, and vice versa. Picture three beats, the first two of which are separated by a wide interval so that the refractory period following the second beat is long. Imagine that the third beat comes early—a premature beat. This third beat will take place in the

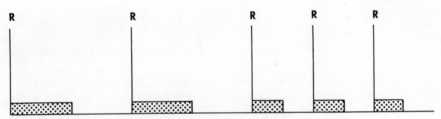

Dotted areas indicate refractory periods following each beat.
Note that the refractory period shortens as the rate increases, and vice-versa.

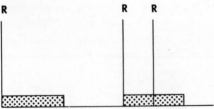

The Ashman phenomenon is the result of this rate-related change in the refractory period. When a short R-R follows a long R-R, the third beat encounters the refractory period set by the preceding long R-R and will be aberrantly conducted.

Fig. 17-6. Ashman phenomenon. (See text.)

prolonged refractory period following the second beat and thus is likely to be aberrantly conducted, since some of the conducting tissues are still in their relative refractory state.

Therefore, when a short R-R interval follows a long R-R interval, look for aberrant intraventricular conduction.

Marriott's criteria of aberrancy versus ectopy

It is not always possible to decide whether a wide QRS complex is the result of aberrant conduction through the ventricular conducting system or of an ectopic ventricular beat. Marriott's studies are the most exhaustive in the attempt to differentiate these two conditions, and they have given much useful information. Recordings of the bundle of His have demonstrated that even with the best criteria it is not always possible to make the distinction between ventricular ectopic firing and ventricular aberration; the diagnosis is still based on statistical likelihood rather than on absolute differentiation. With this limitation in mind, it is well to emphasize and summarize Marriott's criteria:

1. Suspect aberrant intraventricular conduction when a wide ventricular complex is preceded at a conducting distance (.12 to .20 second) by an ectopic P wave.
2. Aberrant conduction, eight times out of ten, will resemble the pattern of right bundle branch block.
3. Because of the Ashman phenomenon, the second beat in a run of rapid beats will be likely to show aberrant conduction. This is because the second beat in a rapid rhythm falls in the relative refractory period of the first beat, which has been set by the longer R-R interval preceding the first beat. A short R-R interval between the first two rapid beats, of course, shortens the refractory period so that subsequent beats are likely to be normally conducted.
4. In lead V_1 an RsR′ pattern is common.
5. The initial deflection of an aberrantly conducted beat is likely to be the same as the initial deflection of the sinus beats in the same lead.

These are not absolute criteria, but when several are detected it is very likely that ventricular aberration, rather than ventricular ectopic firing, is the cause of the wide ventricular complex.

PARASYSTOLE

If the reader will look at most of the ectopic beats illustrated in this text, he will note that the interval from the preceding sinus beat to the ectopic beat is constant (within .10 second). This is because most ectopic beats are actually "triggered" by the passage of the preceding normal sinus beat. Ectopic beats with a constant coupling interval to the preceding sinus beat are referred to as "linked" ectopic beats.

Fig. 17-7 illustrates a different phenomenon. Measure the distance from the sinus beat to the ventricular ectopic beat and note the extreme variation. When the coupling interval of a series of ectopic beats arising in the same focus varies more than .10 second, it is likely that these are *not* triggered by the preceding sinus beat but are in fact the result of independent firing from a parasystolic focus. A parasystolic focus can be thought of as a small pacemaker discharging constantly at a fixed inherent rate and emerging into the myocardium to produce a beat when the tissues are not refractory. It is not coupled to the sinus rhythm in any way.

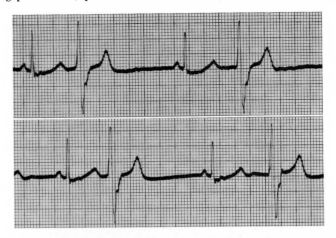

Fig. 17-7. Ventricular parasystole. (See text.)

To prove that a focus is parasystolic, measure the intervals between a series of ectopic beats and see whether or not they reduce to a single common denominator that represents the actual discharge rate of the parasystolic focus.

REFERENCES

Berkman, N., and Lamb, L.: The Wolff-Parkinson-White electrocardiogram: a followup study of five to twenty-eight years, New Engl. J. Med. **278**:492-494, 1968.

Marriott, H. J. L.: Practical electrocardiography, ed. 4, Baltimore, 1968, The Williams & Wilkins Co.

Wolff, L., Parkinson, J., and White, P.: Bundle-branch block with short P-R interval in healthy young people prone to paroxysmal tachycardia, Am. Heart J. **5**:685-704, 1930.

18 Problems, practice, and reinforcement: 3

These are very difficult arrhythmias; some of them will tax the most experienced cardiologist. Each poses a problem of prognosis and therapy that can be elucidated only by the correct diagnosis.

PROBLEM 1: A 65-year-old patient who has been taking 0.25 mg of digoxin per day presents with symptoms of weakness and near-collapse. The patient also describes "feelings of fluttering in the heart." The rhythm is recorded (Fig. 18-1).

QUESTIONS:

1. Diagnosis?
2. Cause?
3. Treatment?

ANSWERS:

1. The first three beats show a normal sinus rhythm. The fourth ventricular complex is a premature ventricular beat (PVC). Just ahead of the PVC is a peculiar tall wave that might be a P wave or a T wave. Inspection of the other T waves in this lead shows that this complex must in fact be a P wave, presumably from an ectopic focus. Since the normal P-R interval is about .18 second, this ectopic P wave could not have produced the wide ventricular complex that immediately follows it. The PVC is followed by a normal sinus beat, which again is followed by three large waves resembling the ectopic P wave preceding the PVC. These waves come very rapidly. They are not followed by a ventricular response. Two normal sinus beats complete the second strip.

   In the second strip there are two atrial complexes for each ventricular complex, that is, there is 2:1 block. The atrial rate is about 188, with some slight variation of spacing of the P waves. The diagnosis in the second strip, therefore, is paroxysmal atrial tachycardia with A-V block.

   In the first strip it is clear that there is a run of three ectopic atrial complexes with complete failure of conduction to the ventricles. This is a very short run of paroxysmal atrial tachycardia with block. The short bursts of nonconducted P waves in the first strip simply give the warning that there is an ectopic focus in the atria firing intermittently and, further, that there is failure of conduction into the A-V node. This is the classic combination of findings in digitalis-induced paroxysmal atrial tachycardia with A-V block.

2. The cause of the rhythm is clearly digitalis intoxication, presumably associated with low potassium.

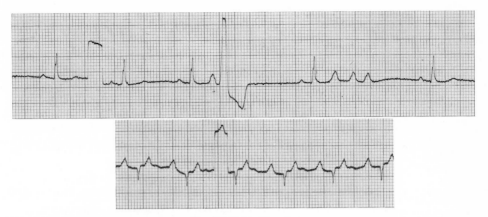

Fig. 18-1. Problem 1.

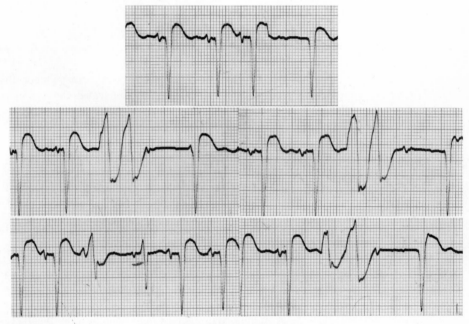

Fig. 18-2. Problem 2.

3. Treatment consists of intravenous infusion of potassium.

    CAUTION: Remember to look for the earliest sign of atrial ectopic firing with any kind of A-V block when considering the possibility of digitalis intoxication.

PROBLEM 2: A 65-year-old patient in the coronary care unit following an anterior infarction manifests an irregular rhythm with frequent pauses and many premature beats. The monitor shows the pattern recorded here (separate strips recorded a few seconds apart) (Fig. 18-2).

QUESTIONS:

1. How many "causes of pauses" can you see in this electrocardiogram?
2. Is the A-V node diseased or is it functioning normally?
3. What specific therapy is needed, and why?

ANSWERS:

1. In the top strip the first two beats are normal sinus beats; the third beat is a premature atrial beat. In the P wave of the premature atrial beat you notice a notch representing another premature P wave, which in this case is not conducted to the ventricles—it is completely blocked. Thus the first "cause of pause" is a blocked premature atrial beat. The last beat on the top strip is an A-V junctional escape beat.

   In the second row, the first two beats are normal sinus beats; the third and fourth are PVC's. After the two PVC's a blocked P wave is noted. This is the second "cause of pause"—there is *concealed conduction* from the two PVC's up into the A-V node that has left the A-V conducting tissues refractory. As a result, the P wave following the PVC's is blocked. The last beat in this strip is another junctional escape beat. On the right-hand side of the second strip this phenomenon is repeated: two PVC's are followed by a blocked P wave.

   In the third strip on the left, two normal sinus beats are followed by a premature P wave. This is followed, at a very short interval, by a wide QRS complex that seems to be "intermediate" in shape between the PVC's noted in other parts of the strip and the normal QRS complexes. Thus a fusion beat is present; the premature P wave partially penetrated the ventricles at the same time that the ventricular ectopic focus fired. Part of ventricular activation, therefore, is "from above, down" through the normal path and part is from below, from the ventricular ectopic beat.

   The third "cause of pause" in this tracing is a simple postectopic pause following the premature atrial beat. (Note the slightly different shape of P and ventricular complex in the first sinus beat following the pause.)

   In the right-hand side of the lower strip the second "cause of pause" is noted: concealed conduction from two PVC's with subsequent blocking of a P wave and a junctional escape beat.

2. It is likely that that A-V conducting tissues are diseased. Blocking of P waves immediately after two PVC's, with concealed conduction into the A-V node, is not unusual and does not necessarily mean that the A-V conducting tissues are abnormal. On the other hand, the blocked P wave following the two PVC's (right-hand side of middle strip) comes long enough after the PVC's so that the A-V conducting tissues should have recovered. The fact that they have not suggests some disease of these tissues, either in the A-V node or in the upper bundle branch system.

3. If the patient is taking digitalis the drug should be stopped for two reasons: there is ventricular ectopic firing, and there is evidence of A-V conduction failure. Since the ventricular ectopic beats are blocking subsequent P waves because of concealed conduction, eradication of the PVC's is an essential part of treatment. If the patient is not taking digitalis, treatment of the PVC's with lidocaine would improve the basic rhythm. Blocked premature atrial complexes (as noted in the top strip) are a characteristic of digitalis toxicity and should always arouse suspicion.

PROBLEM 3: A patient with chronic arteriosclerotic heart disease who has been known to have had an "irregular heart rhythm" for some years describes weakness, a sensation of "pounding of the heart," and some nausea. The rhythm strips shown in Fig. 18-3 are recorded.

QUESTIONS:

1. What is the basic arrhythmia?
2. Is complete A-V block present or not?
3. Treatment?

ANSWERS:

1. The basic rhythm is atrial fibrillation. Ventricular rhythm is represented by a series of narrow QRS complexes, followed at a fixed coupling interval by wide, bizarre, ventricular complexes. Initial diagnosis is atrial fibrillation with ventricular bigeminy.

2. Conduction to the ventricles from fibrillating atria always produces an irregular rhythm. The narrow QRS complexes obviously originate from some point above the bifurcation of the bundle branches and may be conducted down from the atria. The first step is to see whether these narrow complexes are regular or irregular. Initially they appear irregular in spacing, which would lead to a tentative diagnosis of simple atrial fibrillation. Closer inspection reveals two consistent patterns or configurations of the narrow ventricular complexes. The first, third, fourth, fifth, and sixth narrow complexes in the top strip and the first, second, and last narrow ventricular complexes in the second strip all have an RSR' configuration. Other ventricular complexes have an

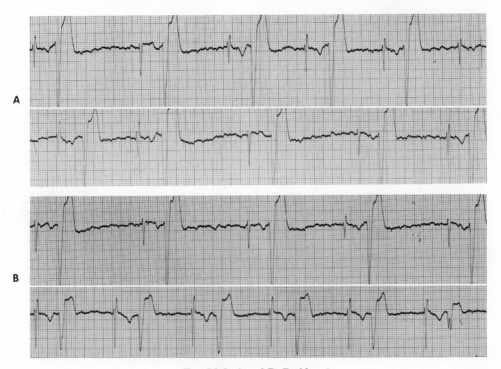

Fig. 18-3. A and **B**, Problem 3.

"rS." The spacing of the RSR′ complexes in the top right strip is absolutely regular.

This raises the possibility that there may be *two* junctional pacemakers firing, each setting its own rhythm and each with its own configuration. This further raises the possibility that there may be *no* conduction from atria to ventricles. *Proof:* Inspect the strips. Note that wherever the RSR′ complex is seen, there is an absolutely regular rhythm with an R-R interval of 168 msec. On the other hand, wherever the rS type of complex is present, another regular rhythm with an interval of 232 msec is noted.

Conclusion: There is complete A-V block; there is no conduction from the fibrillating atria to the ventricles. The ventricular rhythm is being set by *two* junctional pacemakers, each with its own rhythm and its own characteristic QRS configuration. One junctional pacemaker is much slower than the other.

Further conclusion: Digitalis toxicity is almost certainly present.

3. Withdraw digitalis and possibly pace the ventricles if the patient's cardiac output is compromised. If the ventricular ectopic beating presents a problem, diphenylhydantoin may be used.

PROBLEM 4: A 70-year-old patient with calcific valvular disease has been taking 0.25 mg of digoxin daily for over a year. He presents with acute dyspnea, near collapse, and a blood pressure of 80/60. The strip shown in Fig. 18-4, *A*, is recorded in the coronary care unit.

QUESTIONS:

1. Basic rhythm?
2. Cause?
3. Treatment?

ANSWERS:

1. In Fig. 18-4, *A*, a regular ventricular rhythm interruped by two ventricular ectopic beats is apparent. The spacing of the narrow ventricular complexes seems irregular, but this is an optical illusion (try measuring with calipers). There are no regular P waves. Some small definite complexes are noticed at varying intervals between the QRS complexes; these are presumably atrial complexes of some sort.

A step in logic: Atrial complexes are present but have a varying relation-

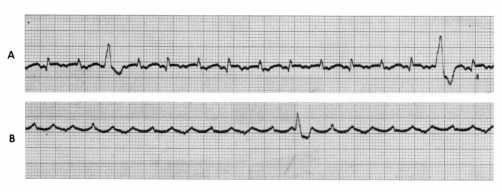

Fig. 18-4. A and **B**, Problem 4.

ship to the ventricular complexes. The ventricular complexes are *regular*. The conclusion, therefore, is that the ventricular complexes cannot be related to the atrial complexes. A junctional tachycardia must be present, while some rapid atrial rhythm is noted at the same time.

Fig. 18-4, *B*, taken during carotid sinus pressure, reveals the source of the atrial rhythm—atrial flutter. Three ventricular escape beats are noted on this tracing.

2. The cause of the rhythm is obviously digitalis toxicity. Junctional tachycardia is a common manifestation of digitalis toxicity. The junctional rhythm is so rapid that none of the atrial impulses would have a chance to penetrate to the ventricles, even if the A-V node were healthy. There is no opportunity, therefore, to draw any conclusions about the functional state of the A-V conducting tissues. One can state only that a junctional tachycardia is present, together with an atrial flutter.

3. Withdraw digitalis and check electrolytes. If potassium is depressed, replace potassium intravenously, as in paroxysmal atrial tachycardia with block.

PROBLEM 5: A patient has recently had an anterior myocardial infarction. His heart rate has gradually been speeding until this rhythm strip is recorded (Fig. 18-5).

QUESTIONS:
1. Rhythm?
2. Significance?
3. Treatment?

ANSWERS:
1. The basic rhythm seems to be a sinus tachycardia. The P-R interval seems short, but this is an artifact of the monitor lead; part of the atrial complex is actually hidden in the baseline. Except for the two pauses, the rate is fairly regular but it does vary somewhat (between 136 and 150). The gradual buildup of rate and the variation in rhythm distinguish this sinus tachycardia from a true paroxysmal atrial tachycardia. After the fourth ventricular complex a P wave is blocked; the same thing happens after the eleventh complex.

Blocking of occasional P waves, without preceding P-R prolongation, is Mobitz Type 2 block.

2. Mobitz Type 2 block implies a much worse prognosis than Mobitz Type 1 (Wenckebach). In association with anterior myocardial infarction, this suggests that the left anterior descending branch of the left coronary artery has been occluded near its origin. The probable mortality is about 75%. The site of the block is likely to be in the upper bundle branch system.

3. A transvenous pacemaker should be inserted at once and personnel should be prepared for a catastrophe, which is very likely to follow.

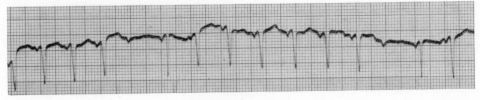

Fig. 18-5. Problem 5.

PROBLEM 6: A patient with severe chronic, obstructive lung disease is seen in the emergency room, where he is noted to be cyanotic, severely dyspneic, and complaining of weakness and "pounding of the heart" (Fig. 18-6).

QUESTIONS:

1. Diagnosis?
2. Cause?
3. Treatment?

ANSWERS:

1. Notice the multiple P waves with varying shapes at irregular spacing. This is a typical chaotic atrial rhythm. There are multiple atrial pacemakers firing, and many of the atrial impulses are blocked. Sometimes atrial impulses seem to be conducted to the ventricles, while at other times, as in the middle of the top strip, there seem to be occasional junctional beats. The majority of the ventricular impulses here are conducted from a preceding P wave and are frequently followed by a blocked P wave.
2. Chronic, obstructive lung disease with severe arterial hypoxemia is the common cause of this arrhythmia. Digitalis toxicity may aggravate the condition.
3. Correct the hypoxemia. Digitalis will usually do more harm than good, and initial efforts should all be directed toward improving ventilation. The prognosis of this arrhythmia is very grave. When it appears in a patient with chronic obstructive lung disease, it implies extremely severe disease and a short life expectancy.

PROBLEM 7: Digitalization has been started in a patient with congestive heart failure caused by rheumatic heart disease. This rhythm appears on a monitor strip (Fig. 18-7).

QUESTIONS:

1. Basic rhythm?
2. Condition of A-V conducting tissues?
3. Treatment?

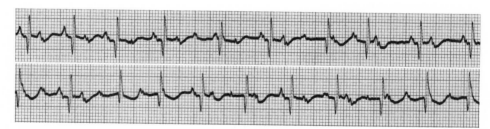

Fig. 18-6. Problem 6.

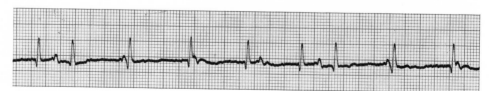

Fig. 18-7. Problem 7.

ANSWERS:

1. The basic rhythm is interference-dissociation with occasional captures. Notice the first, third, and fourth ventricular complexes. These clearly represent an A-V junctional rhythm; so do the fifth, sixth, eighth, and ninth beats. The second and seventh beats are premature. These beats are preceded by a P wave at a distance of .22 second; they represent *capture* of the rhythm by the S-A node. Look carefully; the other sinus P waves can be seen, although often they are hidden by the junctional beats.

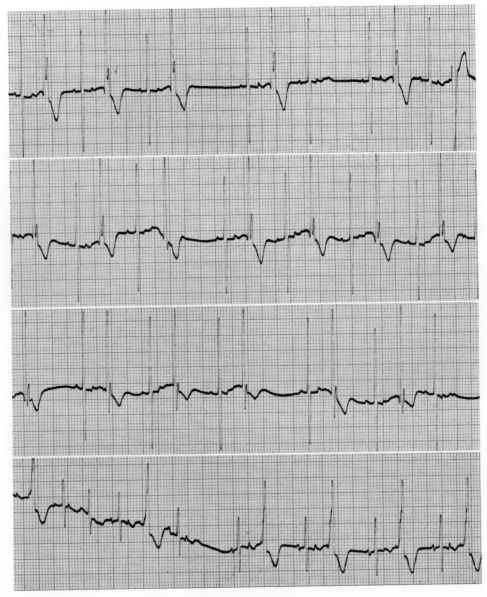

Fig. 18-8. Problem 8.

2. The A-V conducting tissues are capable of functioning normally, as shown in the two capture beats. The reason for the abnormal rhythm is the slow rate of the S-A node, which permits the escape of an interfering junctional pacemaker.

3. Speed the S-A node with atropine. If this is not adequate and if the patient's condition appears critical, atrial pacing should be used.

PROBLEM 8: This tracing was recorded on a newborn infant with evidence of heart failure attributed to myocarditis, type unknown. Digitalis had been administered for 2 days before the rhythm shown here was detected (Fig. 18-8).

QUESTIONS:

1. Rhythm?

2. Clinical significance?

ANSWERS:

1. Reading from left to right across the top strip, a normal sinus beat is followed by a premature beat (the second beat in the strip). This premature complex consists of a P wave followed by a wide QRS with a different configuration and axis from normal. This pattern of a normal sinus beat followed by a premature beat is repeated five times. After the ninth beat, which is a normal sinus beat, there is a premature P wave but no ventricular response.

   The diagnosis so far is normal sinus rhythm with premature atrial beats, aberrantly conducted, forming a bigeminal rhythm. There is one blocked premature atrial beat.

   The twelfth beat is a normal sinus beat. The premature atrial beat following it shows a completely different axis of ventricular activation from the other premature beats. Since the two patterns of aberrant conduction visible are 180 degrees apart in axis, it seems clear that there is fascicular block as the basis of the aberration. Block of the anterior fascicle of the left bundle produces one type of aberrant beat, while block of the posterior or inferior fascicle produces the other. Since the lead shown here is a monitor lead, it is not possible to say which fascicle is blocked in the two types of aberration.

   The same pattern is repeated throughout the tracing. Note the varying P-R interval of the premature beats and the occasional blocked premature atrial beats. Note further that after the third ventricular complex from the right-hand end in the third strip there seems to be two atrial complexes in rapid succession.

   The essential elements of this arrhythmia therefore are:
   a. Multiple premature atrial beats, usually forming a bigeminal rhythm
   b. Varying degree of A-V block of the premature beats
   c. Aberrant conduction within the ventricles manifested during the premature beats

2. The first two elements speak strongly for digitalis toxicity. The drug was stopped and the rhythm became normal.

PROBLEM 9: This tracing was recorded on a 33-year-old patient without history of heart disease who was seen at the emergency room for severe alcoholic intoxication (Fig. 18-9).

QUESTIONS:

1. Basic rhythm?

2. Cause of change in configuration of ventricular complexes in various parts of the tracing?
3. Cause of change in configuration of P waves in various parts of the tracing?
4. Significance?

ANSWERS:

1. Basic rhythm is sinus tachycardia with periods of A-V junctional rhythm. The second and third strips both start with a regular rhythm, a rate of 88, and no apparent P waves. The QRS complexes are narrow. The diagnosis of A-V junctional rhythm is established. In the midportion of the second and third strips and in the left- and right-hand side of the bottom strip, clear-cut sinus rhythm is present.

2. A curious change in QRS configuration is noted between the A-V junctional rhythm and the sinus rhythm. During the periods of A-V junctional rhythm an initial negative deflection is noted in the QRS complex, which resembles a "coronary" Q wave. This initial negative deflection is not present during the periods of sinus rhythm. Obviously, what seems to be a Q wave is in fact a retrograde P wave, indicating that the A-V junctional impulse traveling up reaches the atria just before the impulse traveling down reaches the ventricles. The appearance of a coronary Q wave is simply an artifact, and the disappearance of this complex when antegrade conduction from the sinus node resumes clearly establishes these peculiar waves as retrograde P waves rather than Q waves.

3. An interesting change in P wave configuration illustrates the phenomenon of intra-atrial fusion. Notice the second complex in the top lead: this is clearly junctional, with a deep, retrograde P wave immediately preceding the ventricular complex. In the third complex the retrograde P wave is not so prominent (it is only about half as deep); in the fourth complex, there is an upright P wave that is continued for the next six beats. The same sequence is noted in the fifth, sixth, and seventh beats in the second strip. The fifth beat,

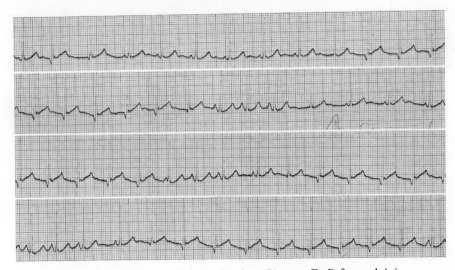

Fig. 18-9. Problem 9. (Courtesy Dr. Jerry Bierman, Ft. Defiance, Ariz.)

like those preceding it, has a deep, retrograde P wave; the sixth has a much shallower retrograde P wave, and the seventh P wave is upright. The explanation for this progressive change is that the retrograde impulse from the junction meets the antegrade impulse from the S-A node and a fusion-type of P wave results. This is analogous to the fusion QRS's described earlier in this book.

4. This disorder of rhythm has no intrinsic significance. The important point here is to differentiate between the retrograde atrial complexes during the junctional rhythm and a coronary Q wave, a decision of considerable significance in planning the patient's care.

PROBLEM 10: Lead V₆ was recorded in a patient with symptoms and signs of myocardial infarction (Fig. 18-10).

QUESTIONS:

1. Diagnosis?
2. Significance?

ANSWERS:

1. The second full beat on the top strip shows the typical configuration of left bundle branch block; the QRS is .14 second wide and there is no septal Q wave. The first beat, however, is much narrower, the total width being about .11 second. The fourth beat manifests complete left bundle branch block, the fifth is narrower, and so on throughout the tracing. In other words, there are alternating wide and narrow ventricular complexes. Complete left bundle branch block is present in the first full complex, while incomplete block in the left bundle branch system is noted in the second; in the second full beat and in every alternate beat thereafter, there is some degree of penetration into the left bundle branch system, even though activation is slower than normal. In the beats with wide QRS complexes the left bundle obviously does not conduct at all. There is, therefore, 2:1 block in a part of the left bundle branch system, probably in one of the two fascicles. REMEMBER: Any form of block seen in the A-V conducting system can also be seen within the bundle branches.

2. The significance of this observation is that the left bundle branch is not completely "dead" functionally; a part of the left bundle branch system

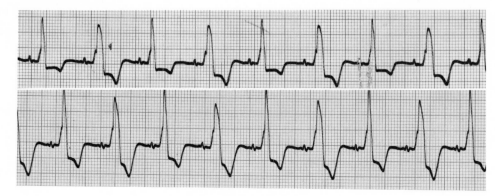

Fig. 18-10. Problem 10.

simply has a very prolonged refractory period that produces left bundle branch block on every other beat or a 2:1 block within the left bundle branch system. The appearance of any kind of bundle branch block in a patient with a myocardial infarct is a very grave sign and preparation should be made for some catastrophe, quite possibly a standstill.

PROBLEM 11: A patient who is taking 0.25 mg of digoxin per day describes a feeling of weakness and near collapse (Fig. 18-11).

QUESTIONS:

1. Basic rhythm?
2. Cause?
3. Treatment?

ANSWERS:

1. The basic rhythm here is paroxysmal atrial tachycardia with A-V block, with one ventricular ectopic beat. The strip starts with a P wave, followed at a prolonged distance (.24 second) by a narrow QRS complex. The next P wave is again followed by a QRS complex but at a still longer distance; this progressive prolongation is noted with the third and fourth P waves, which seem to "disappear" into the preceding ventricular complexes as the P-R lengthens. The fifth and sixth P waves are hidden in the ventricular complexes; the sixth P wave is blocked and a pause follows, characteristic of the end of a Wenckebach cycle. After the fifth ventricular complex, a P wave is again noted, which is conducted to the ventricles, and a second Wenckebach cycle starts. This second Wenckebach cycle runs through seven atrial complexes and six ventricular responses before a P wave is blocked. A PVC is noted after the second Wenckebach cycle.

2. The cause is almost certainly digitalis toxicity, accentuated by low serum potassium.

3. Treatment consists of replacing potassium.

PROBLEM 12: A patient presents in the emergency room with a rapid, regular pulse that is described as having appeared abruptly, accompanied by sensations of "pounding in the chest" and weakness. The tracing is recorded (Fig. 18-12).

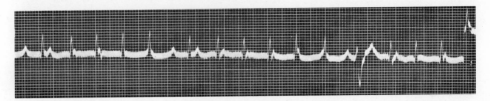

Fig. 18-11. Problem 11.

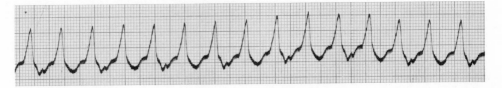

Fig. 18-12. Problem 12.

QUESTIONS:

1. Differential diagnosis?
2. Treatment?

ANSWERS:

1. Wide ventricular complexes are noted at a rate of 150; the rhythm is regular. Differential diagnosis, therefore, includes paroxysmal atrial tachycardia with bundle branch block, paroxysmal junctional tachycardia with bundle branch block, and paroxysmal ventricular tachycardia.

   Note that after every alternate ventricular complex there is a retrograde P wave appearing as a notch in the T wave. These could not possibly be antegrade atrial complexes, since they are noted only every other complex at a fixed distance after the QRS. Since the ventricular rhythm is regular and since every alternate ventricular complex is *not* preceded by an atrial complex, it would be impossible for this to be atrial tachycardia.

   Differential diagnosis here lies between junctional tachycardia with bundle branch block and paroxysmal ventricular tachycardia. It is not possible from this tracing alone to make the distinction. If previous tracings were available that showed ventricular ectopic beats with a configuration identical to the ventricular complexes on this tracing, it would be helpful.

2. Use carotid sinus stimulation. If the rhythm is A-V junctional, the vagal stimulation may end the tachycardia; if it is ventricular, there will be no effect. If carotid sinus stimulation is ineffective, *treat the more dangerous possibility—that is, treat this arrhythmia as if it were a proved paroxysmal ventricular tachycardia.* Use lidocaine, procainamide, or quinidine; these drugs will do no harm if the rhythm is actually an A-V junctional tachycardia. Quinidine is sometimes effective in junctional as well as in ventricular tachycardias. *On the other hand, the preferred treatment for A-V junctional tachycardia, digitalis, may very well be lethal if the rhythm is actually ventricular tachycardia.*

Part IV
DRUGS AND TECHNIQUE

19 Drugs and dosages

DIGITALIS

Digoxin is probably the most widely used form of digitalis at this time. It can be administered orally, intravenously, or intramuscularly.

Oral administration. Contrary to common belief, it is not necessary to give a large single initial dose of digoxin to achieve rapid oral digitalization. An initial dose of 0.25 mg, or at the most 0.5 mg, followed by doses of 0.25 mg every 6 hours probably gives as efficient oral digitalization as needed. Total dose will vary two- or threefold, depending on age, renal function, body mass, and so on. The "average" digitalizing dose of 1.25 mg in the first 24 hours is only an approximation. Always titrate the drug against the patient's response in terms of pulse rate, diuresis, symptomatic improvement, and the like.

SLOW DIGITALIZATION. Contrary to pharmacologists, many older clinicians avowed that "slow digitalization works!" They were absolutely right. Marcus and associates have demonstrated that a maintenance dose of digoxin given daily produces the same effect in about 1 week as any of the more intensive modes of administration. Thus 0.25 mg of digoxin daily accomplishes full digitalization within approximately 1 week, which is ample for the needs of many patients.

Intravenous administration. Three warnings should be given here:
1. Intravenous digitalis preparations of any kind are dangerous.
2. Intravenous administration of digitalis compounds often is not necessary.
3. Intravenous digitalis preparations always should be given *very slowly;* for example, 0.25 mg of digoxin should never be given in less than 15 minutes.

I have seen two deaths from minimal doses of digitalis preparations given intravenously. This is a poison, remember, for which there is no immediate antidote.

Intravenous administration of digoxin and other digitalis preparations is much too common, and the drug is almost always given too rapidly. If the drug is administered intravenously in less than 15 minutes, toxic levels accumulate at the cellular interface, frequently with disastrous results. Many readers of this book will doubtless be thinking that they have given intravenous digitalis quite rapidly many times without killing anybody. I can only say they are simply waiting for the law of averages to catch up with them.

A conservative schedule of intravenous administration, but one with a sound basis in pharmacology, is to administer a dose of 0.25 mg of digoxin initially over 15 minutes. Repeat in 2 hours, if needed, and then in 4 hours, adjusting subsequent doses until the desired effect is obtained.

Intramuscular administration. Intramuscular digoxin has the advantage of safety for patients who cannot take oral medication. The action of intramuscular digoxin is about equivalent to that administered orally. There is considerable discomfort attendent upon the injection, but it is a good substitute for the oral route when this is impractical.

Maintenance dose. Maintenance dose of digoxin will be 0.25 mg per day or 0.125 mg per day *or less* in older patients or those with impaired renal function.

DIGITALIS LEAF

Digitalis leaf, which is a mixture of several glycosides, reaches an appreciable level of action in 2 to 5 hours when given orally. Maximum effect is noted within 24 hours, usually somewhere between 12 and 16 hours. Excretion is prolonged, taking about 14 days.

As a rule of thumb, a dose of 100 mg per 10 pounds of lean body weight given over the first 24 to 36 hours works out surprisingly well for rapid digitalization with digitalis leaf.

Maintenance dose. The maintenance dose is 100 mg per day.

DIGITOXIN

Digitoxin is the most slowly excreted of all digitalis compounds (excretion time is 14 to 21 days). It is most useful in patients with impaired renal function, since excretion and metabolism are independent of renal function.

Oral administration. The "digitalizing" dose is 1.2 mg given in divided doses over 24 to 36 hours. The initial dose may be 0.2 to 0.4 mg followed by 0.2 mg every 4 hours until digitalization has been achieved, as judged by the response of the patient.

Intravenous administration. Digitoxin may be given intravenously in the same doses. Remember the precautions about *slow* administration!

Maintenance dose. An average maintenance dose of digitoxin is 0.1 mg per day, although there is considerable individual variation.

DESLANOSIDE

Deslanoside is a later version of the preparation formerly known as "lanatoside C." The advantage of this drug is rapid onset of action. After intravenous administration, an effect is apparent within about 5 minutes, with a peak of 30 to 40 minutes.

The initial dose is 0.4 to 0.6 mg. Subsequent doses are 0.2 to 0.4 mg every 2 hours.

It is difficult to maintain patients using the oral form of this drug. The only real indications for its use are conditions in which acute digitalis effect is needed or in which prolonged use of the drug is not anticipated (that is, in the conversion of paroxysmal atrial tachycardia).

QUINIDINE

First, if possible, check for quinidine sensitivity with a test dose of 50 mg.

Oral administration. For conversion of atrial fibrillation, atrial flutter, or ventricular tachycardia, give 200 mg orally at 2-hour intervals or 100 mg hourly. After about 10 to 12 hours the serum level of quinidine will have reached a plateau where it will remain reasonably constant unless the dose is increased. After 12 hours (total of 1 to 2 gm) it is probably best to shift to 0.2 gm every 4 hours, with careful monitoring of quinidine levels, if possible. If conversion is not attained at the end of 24 hours on this schedule, 200 mg every 2 hours may be given during the next two 24-hour periods. This will probably produce a slow rise in the serum quinidine level.

Observe carefully for evidence of toxicity—nausea, vomiting, falling of blood pressure, widening of QRS complex, or A-V block. Remember that the toxic range of quinidine is 8 to 10 mg/100 ml and that the therapeutic range is probably about 2 to 4 mg/100 ml, although the correlation between therapeutic effect and blood level is not really satisfactory.

Intramuscular administration. Quinidine may be administered intramuscularly when the oral route is not practical. Doses of 100 mg may be injected, using roughly the same dose schedules as indicated for the oral route.

Intravenous administration. Never use intravenous quinidine—it is extremely dangerous!

Maintenance dose. Once conversion of an arrhythmia is attained, a maintenance dose of 200 mg four times a day will usually sustain a sinus rhythm if this is physiologically possible.

Treatment of ventricular ectopic beats. The maintenance dose of quinidine, 200 to 400 mg four times per day, will usually produce maximum effect.

PROCAINAMIDE (PRONESTYL)

Procainamide may be administered orally, intramuscularly, or intravenously.

Intravenous administration. Intravenous procainamide is extremely useful in the treatment of ventricular tachyarrhythmias, that is, ventricular tachycardia or repetitive ventricular firing. The drug is given by intravenous drip. Dissolve 1 gm of procainamide in 500 to 1,000 ml of appropriate solution and drip under constant monitoring and observation. *The chief danger associated with intravenous procainamide is an abrupt drop in blood pressure.* When administering procainamide intravenously, always connect with a Y tube to a reservoir of a pressor amine (such as levarterenol).

The rate of drip may be rapid initially (about 120 drops per minute) and may be slowed when the arrhythmia is corrected or when blood pressure begins to fall. The 1-gm dose may be repeated two or three times in a 24-hour period.

The intravenous method is the most dangerous method of administering procainamide and should be reserved for very grave emergencies. Intramuscular or oral use is almost always preferable.

Intramuscular administration. Intramuscular administration of 0.25 gm of procainamide at 2-hour intervals, or 0.5 gm at 4-hour intervals, achieves satisfactory blood levels promptly and is probably as effective as the intravenous route for all practical purposes. A total dose of 3 to 4 gm may be given by this route in 24 hours.

Oral administration. Recent evidence suggests that much larger oral doses of procainamide must be used than were formerly thought necessary. In an acutely ill patient, give 0.5 to 1.0 gm every 2 hours; for less severe arrhythmias give 0.25 to 0.50 gm every 4 hours. For prophylactic or maintenance dose, use 0.25 to 0.50 gm four times a day.

LIDOCAINE

Intravenous administration

BOLUS ADMINISTRATION. For ventricular tachyarrhythmias (ventricular tachycardia or repetitive ventricular ectopic firing), 50 to 75 mg of lidocaine is injected rapidly as a bolus. This can be repeated three or four times over a 10-minute period.

INTRAVENOUS DRIP. Dissolve 1 gm of lidocaine in 500 to 1,000 ml of solution. The drip is administered so that the patient receives 1 to 4 mg per minute. Watch for toxic effects, that is, evidence of convulsive movements or twitchings.

Intramuscular administration. Recently, attempts have been made to administer lidocaine intramuscularly. Satisfactory blood levels have been achieved by this route, and intramuscular administration may come to be an accepted mode of treatment, particularly for outpatient emergency use.

DIPHENYLHYDANTOIN (DILANTIN)

Diphenylhydantoin has been reported to be beneficial in the treatment of atrial tachyarrhythmias, but in my experience this application of the drug has been disappointing. Diphenylhydantoin may be given orally or intravenously. Bigger and associates, in a classic study on the use of this drug, defined the effective plasma level of diphenylhydantoin in the range between 10 and 18 $\mu g/ml$. These workers pointed out that a critical effective plasma level was essential before any antiarrhythmic activity of the drug could be demonstrated.

Intravenous administration. As recommended by Bigger, give successive doses of 50 to 100 mg of diphenylhydantoin every 5 minutes until the arrhythmia is abolished, until 1,000 mg has been given, or until undesirable effects appear. NOTE: Intravenous diphenylhydantoin has been fatal. *Close electrocardiographic and clinical monitoring is essential.*

Oral administration. A loading dose would be 1,000 mg in divided doses on the first day, 500 to 600 mg on the second and third days, and subsequent maintenance doses of 400 to 500 mg per day.

WARNING: Even when diphenylhydantoin is given with these precautions, it remains a dangerous drug. I know of two deaths that followed intravenous administration of diphenylhydantoin given with this exact protocol. *Balance the risk of the treatment against the risk of the arrhythmia.*

EDROPHONIUM (TENSILON)

Edrophonium is a parasympathomimetic drug. The effect of edrophonium on an arrhythmia is exactly the same as the effect of vagal stimulation by carotid sinus massage, except that the drug is more potent and the effect is more sustained. Edrophonium has two specific uses: (1) It is used to treat paroxysmal supraventricular tachycardia. (2) It aids in the diagnosis of atrial flutter or paroxysmal atrial tachycardia with A-V block.

In these arrhythmias, edrophonium is useful since it slows conduction through the A-V node and permits diagnostic evaluation of the atrial complexes. If a patient with atrial flutter, for example, does not show A-V nodal delay with carotid sinus massage, 5 mg of edrophonium may be injected intravenously. If the drug alone does not produce adequate slowing, carotid sinus massage may be added, and a cumulative vagal effect will frequently slow conduction through the A-V node sufficiently to permit diagnostic evaluation of atrial complexes.

Contraindications to the use of edrophonium are the same as to any parasympathomimetic drug—bronchial asthma, peptic ulcer, and the like.

BRETYLIUM TOSYLATE

This drug was the subject of much premature and overenthusiastic evaluation. At this point it probably has no place in the armamentarium of the clinician.

BETA-ADRENERGIC BLOCKING AGENTS

The reader may have wondered at the absence of any mention of beta-adrenergic blocking agents in this book. The omission has been deliberate. Beta-adrenergic blocking agents, that is, propranolol and practolol, are extremely useful drugs in the treatment of angina pectoris. Their use in the treatment of arrhythmias has been premature, overenthusiastic, frequently ill advised, and sometimes lethal.

There are two reasons for these emphatic comments.

1. Beta-adrenergic blocking agents exert a powerful, negative inotropic effect. In the presence of a compromised myocardium the use of these agents may depress cardiac output past a point of no return, with fatal results.
2. The vast majority of arrhythmias can be treated by safer and more effective means.

Probably the major indication for the use of beta-adrenergic blocking drugs in treating arrhythmias is the prevention of recurrent supraventricular tachycardias associated with the Wolff-Parkinson-White syndrome. *Always begin with small doses, always increase gradually, and never administer the drug intravenously.* (I have seen at least one death follow the intravenous administration of propranolol.)

Recurrent paroxysmal supraventricular tachycardia in patients with otherwise healthy hearts is another legitimate indication for the use of beta-blockade. This is particularly true in young patients, who will be substantially free of the risk of covert coronary artery disease. In the absence of any evidence of heart disease, doses of propranolol may be increased more rapidly than would otherwise be the case. (Patients with angina pectoris, for example, often tolerate doses of several hundred milligrams per day.) The rule of small initial doses, of the order of 10 mg three times per day increased gradually with careful observation for evidence of heart failure, is still sound. *If the physician is not expert in analysis of heart sounds, including gallop sounds, and in inspection of jugular venous pulsations, he should not be prescribing large doses of beta-blocking agents.* (This may all sound ultraconservative, but I have strong views about needless death and suffering produced by medical meddling.)

Oral administration. Give 10 mg three times a day; increase very gradually to 20 or 30 mg three times per day. If the patient is known to have any type of heart disease, watch carefully for evidence of failure.

ATROPINE

Atropine has two uses in the treatment of cardiac arrhythmias: (1) It speeds the rate of firing of the S-A node. (2) It accelerates A-V nodal conduction.

Intravenous or subcutaneous administration. Atropine is given in doses of 0.50 to 1 mg.

Oral administration. In the rare patient who will need prolonged antivagal medication, it is best to use tincture of belladonna. The danger of accidental ingestion of a lethal dose when a patient is given a large number of atropine tablets is very great. Tincture of belladonna, on the other hand, is so bitter that it would be almost impossible to ingest a dangerous dose. A normal dose of tincture of belladonna is 10 drops in one-half glass of water three times a day. The dose may be increased to 15 drops, depending on the patient's response.

Contraindications. Remember to check for glaucoma and to be particularly cautious in the elderly patient who may have bladder obstruction.

REFERENCES

Bigger, J. T., Schmidt, D. H., and Kutt, H.: Relationship between the plasma level of diphenylhydantoin sodium and its cardiac artiarrhythmic effects, Circulation **38**:363, 1968.

Ewy, G.: Digitalis therapy in the geriatric patient, Drug Ther. **2**:36-49, 1972.

Ewy, G. A., and others: Digoxin metabolism in obesity, Circulation **44**:810-814, 1971.

Gamble, O., and Cohn, K.: Effect of propranolol, procainamide, and lidocaine on ventricular automaticity and reentry in experimental myocardial infarction, Circulation **46**:498-506, 1972.

Gettes, L.: The electrophysiologic effects of antiarrhythmic drugs, Am. J. Cardiol. **28**:526-535, 1971.

Stone, N., Klein, M., and Lown, B.: Diphenylhydantoin in the prevention of recurring ventricular tachycardia, Circulation **43**:420-427, 1971.

Weisse, A., and others: Relative effectiveness of three antiarrhythmic agents in the treatment of ventricular arrhythmias in experimental acute myocardial ischemia, Am. Heart J. **81**:503-510, 1971.

20 Pacers and pacing

The subject of pacers and pacing could fill several books—in fact, it does. For practical purposes, the clinician needs to know several sets of facts.

INDICATIONS FOR PERMANENT PACING

A permanent pacer should be implanted in the following patients:
1. All patients with acquired third-degree block. The congenital form of complete A-V block is surprisingly benign, and although pacing may be required to increase cardiac output, Stokes-Adams attacks are much less common than in the acquired type. Some cardiologists recommend waiting for a first Stokes-Adams episode before pacing; this is a legitimate difference of opinion and the answer is not yet clear.
2. Patients with chronic second-degree A-V block with Stokes-Adams episodes
3. Patients with bifascicular block with syncope suggestive of Stokes-Adams episodes. With complete right bundle branch block and block of either of the two fascicles of the left bundle, there is at least a 16% chance of complete failure of A-V conduction with long periods of asystole.
4. Patients with the sick sinus syndrome who suffer incapacitating episodes of vertigo or syncope

Indications for temporary pacing

Insertion of a temporary ventricular pacer is indicated in:
1. Anterior myocardial infarction with any degree of A-V block more severe than minimal P-R prolongation
2. Inferior or posterior myocardial infarction with second or third-degree A-V block

Temporary atrial pacing is often useful in the presence of A-V junctional or idioventricular rhythms to restore atrial augmentation of cardiac output in critically ill patients. In this group of patients, atrial pacing may also serve to increase the heart rate to optimal levels when the sinus rate is very slow and when the rate of the escape ectopic rhythm is not adequate for maximum cardiac output.

Atrial pacing may be indicated in patients with severe sick sinus syndrome associated with myocardial infarction or myocardial ischemic episodes, when maximum output is necessary, and when medical therapy does not produce a satisfactory response.

INSERTING A TEMPORARY TRANSVENOUS PACEMAKER

This is a skill that any physician caring for cardiac patients should have at his disposal. Here is a simple protocol.

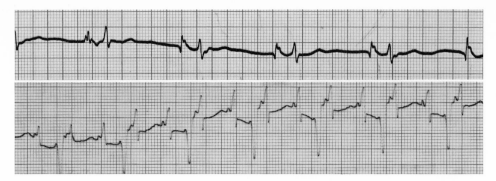

Fig. 20-1. Atrial complexes recorded from within the right atrium. Top strip: Normal sinus rhythm. Note that atrial complexes are larger than ventricular. Second strip: Atrial tachycardia with 2:1 A-V block. The atrial complexes appear at a rate of 148.

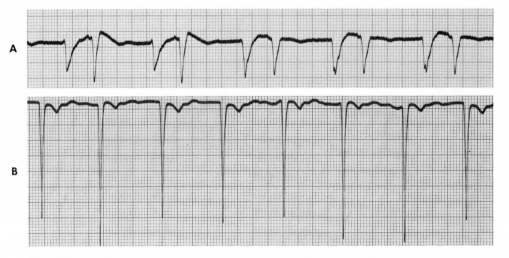

Fig. 20-2. A, Electrocardiogram recorded from within right atrium. Note huge negative atrial complexes. **B,** Electrocardiogram recorded from within right ventricle. Atrial complexes almost disappear; ventricular complexes become huge.

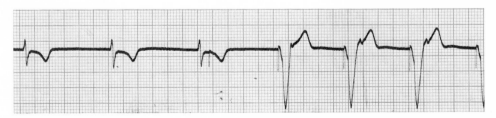

Fig. 20-3. Recognition of pacing from right ventricle. First three complexes are supraventricular; subsequent complexes are wide and are preceded by a pacemaker artifact. Complexes produced by pacing from the right ventricle will have a left bundle branch block configuration. Since these are in fact ventricular ectopic beats, they will always be at least .12 second wide.

Insertion site. The safest site for insertion of a temporary pacemaker is the median basilic vein. Subclavian vein puncture or jugular puncture may be used, but both approaches are relatively dangerous. Puncture of the subclavian artery, with death from massive hemothorax; puncture of the carotid, with uncontrollable bleeding and cerebral complications; and pneumothorax are the complications to be feared. (None of these accompanies the use of an arm vein.)

Monitoring. When the atria are active—when sinus rhythm, atrial fibrillation, or flutter is present—electrocardiographic monitoring offers a simple and very accurate way of following the course of the catheter (Fig. 20-1). When arrest has already taken place, a fluoroscope must be used to place the catheter in the ventricles.

Steps in insertion

1. Using a large-bore needle with a plastic sheath, enter a median basilic vein by cutdown or by puncture.

2. Attach the left and right arm leads of the electrocardiograph to the two poles of the pacing catheter with alligator clips. Set the electrocardiograph on lead I.

3. Thread the catheter up the vein and into the right atrium, watching the electrocardiogram for the characteristic huge atrial complexes when the catheter tip moves from superior vena cava to right atrium (Fig. 20-2, *A*).

4. Float the catheter into the right ventricle, judging arrival in the ventricle by the appearance of huge QRS complexes and the disappearance of the large atrial complexes on the electrocardiogram (Fig. 20-2, *B*).

5. Reconnect the electrocardiograph leads to the patient. Connect the poles of the pacing catheter to a pacer and test for capture of pacing.

Ventricular pacing. A pacer in the right ventricle will produce a wide QRS complex with a left bundle branch block configuration (Fig. 20-3). The pacing tip is in fact producing right ventricular ectopic beats; therefore, look for a pacing spike followed by wide ventricular complexes with a left bundle branch configuration.

If the pacer does not capture the rhythm, increase amperage until the patient notes some discomfort from the impulse. (This will be about 5 ma.) If there is still no capture, manipulate the catheter tip within the ventricle, monitoring again with the electrocardiograph, and try to produce a slight injury current, that is, some elevation of the S-T segment. This usually means that the catheter tip is wedged firmly against the ventricular endocardium and is likely to produce pacing.

Atrial pacing. For atrial pacing try various positions within the right atrium, since there is considerable variability of response. Capture of the rhythm by right atrial pacing is more difficult than ventricular pacing, because the tip of the catheter will not usually be wedged against the atrial wall. Considerable manipulation of the catheter within the atrium will be necessary to capture the rhythm, and there will be frequent periods when capture is lost. However, with careful attention to the rhythm and with proper adjustments, atrial pacing is frequently helpful and sometimes lifesaving.

REFERENCES

DeSanctis, R.: Diagnostic and therapeutic uses of atrial pacing, Circulation **43**:748-761, 1971.
Kaltman, A.: Indications for temporary pacemaker insertion in acute myocardial infarction, Am. Heart J. **81**:837-841, 1971.
Langendorf, R., and Pick, A.: Artificial pacing of the human heart: its contribution to the understanding of the arrhythmias, Am. J. Cardiol. **28**:516-525, 1971.

21 Defibrillators, defibrillation, and cardioversion

Gordon A. Ewy, M.D.*

DEFIBRILLATORS

Imagine a physician prescribing a potent drug. Imagine that, unknown to the physician, the various brands of this drug contained quantities of the active ingredient that varied by as much as 50% in apparently similar tablets. Imagine further that this drug could produce toxic effects of which the physician was ignorant. This is the kind of therapeutic dilemma with which physicians are confronted when prescribing electric therapy for cardiac arrhythmias.

A comparative analysis of direct current defibrillators in use in several hospitals in the United States during 1969 to 1970 revealed marked variations between the amount of energy indicated on the defibrillator dial and the actual amount of energy delivered into a resistive load.[1] For example, at a dial setting of 400 watt-seconds (or joules) the amount of energy delivered into a 50-ohm resistive load varied considerably (Table 1). To deliver 150 watt-seconds of energy, some machines had to be set at 153 watt-seconds and others at increasingly higher energy levels up to a setting of 380 watt-seconds. Several units were not able to deliver 250 watt-seconds of energy against a 50-ohm load, and of those that were, the dial settings varied between 250 and 435 watt-seconds.[1]

Some of the newer defibrillators have dial settings that indicate *delivered* rather than *stored* energy. Some now have two dial readings, one to indicate stored energy and the other to indicate delivered energy against a 50-ohm resistive load.

On most defibrillators, the dial can be set above the 400 watt-second reading. We have referred to this setting as the maximal or "max" setting (Fig. 21-1). At this setting, the amount of energy delivered *above* that delivered at the 400 watt-second setting varied from a few watt-seconds to as high as 173 watt-seconds.[1] Knowing this capability could be helpful if one were unable to defibrillate a patient with the defibrillator dial set at 400 watt-seconds. On the other hand, this increment in delivered energy might cause cardiac damage in other situations. At this writing, few units indicate the amount of delivered energy at maximal setting.

The preceding information should *not* be interpreted to mean that the only important electric parameter in defibrillation is *delivered energy* in watt-seconds—the *electric wave form* and *current* are also important. Before discussing these param-

---

*Teaching Scholar of the American Heart Association.

eters, it might be helpful to digress and review the electronic terminology associated with defibrillator and/or cardioverter discharge.

When stored electric energy is discharged, the resultant current (I) and voltage (V) depends upon the resistance into which the countershock is delivered (Fig. 21-2).

Table 1. Comparative analysis of defibrillators*

Number of machines tested	Defibrillator	Delivered energy in watt-seconds (joules) at dial setting of 400 watt-seconds†
6	General Electric	340
3	Physio-Control Series 70	325
3	Electrodyne D-84-M	305
6	American Optical No. 10646	290
4	Physio-Control Life-Pak	285
2	Mennen-Greatbach	285
4	Burdick DC 150	265
6	Dallons DCM	255
6	Hewlett-Packard 7802B	255
4	American Optical 660-670	240
2	Electronics for Medicine	230
2	Corbin-Farnsworth	225
3	American Optical No. 10525	225
2	Corbin-Farnsworth (Maxcart)	155

*Adapted from Ewy, G. A., Fletcher, R. D., and Ewy, M. D.: Comparative analysis of direct current defibrillators, J. Electrocardiol. **5**:349, 1972.
†Energy delivered into 50-ohm resistive load.

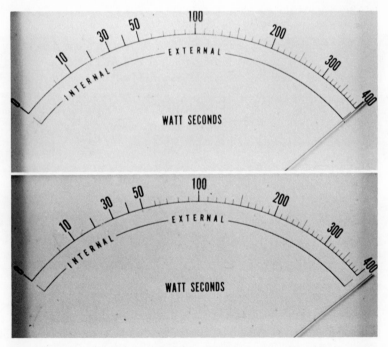

Fig. 21-1. Defibrillator dial. Top: Dial setting at "400 watt-seconds." Bottom: Dial setting at "Max."

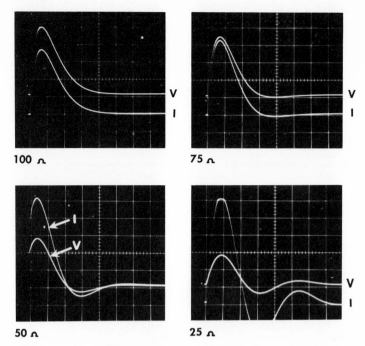

Fig. 21-2. Simultaneous voltage (*V*) and current (*I*) waveforms from a direct current defibrillator discharged into resistive loads of 100, 75, 50, and 25 ohms. Voltage equals 1 kv per division; current equals 10 amp per division, and oscilloscope sweep speed equals 2 msec per division.

It may be helpful to physicians to think of *current* as blood *flow* and *voltage* as blood *pressure*. If, at a constant heart output, a cuff is blown up around the arm, thus increasing the resistance, proximal pressure will increase as distal blood flow decreases. A similar phenomenon occurs with defibrillators: when a fixed energy level (in watt-seconds or joules) is discharged and a high resistance is encountered, the resultant current will be less than if a low resistance is encountered. This concept is important, since Geddes and associates have shown recently that the minimal amount of current required to defibrillate animals is related to body weight.[2] Thus, if one encounters a large patient, it may be necessary to reduce maximally the transthoracic or chest wall resistance in order to deliver an adequate amount of current for defibrillation.

Transthoracic resistance can be reduced by two methods: (1) by using large-size paddle electrodes, and (2) by using an appropriate electrode–chest wall interface. Recent studies have shown that chest wall resistance to direct current countershock decreases with increasing paddle electrode size.[3-5] This also holds true if only one of the two paddle electrodes is larger.[5]

If bare paddles are used on the chest wall, the resistance is high. The resistance can be decreased by using electrode cream or saline-soaked gauze pads; however, the lowest resistance is obtained when electrode paste is used.[5] Table 2 shows the progressive lowering of transthoracic resistance measured with increased paddle sizes and different paddle electrode–chest wall interfaces.[5]

Table 2. Canine transthoracic resistance to DC defibrillator discharge*

Paddle electrode diameter (cm)	Paddle electrode–chest wall interface			
	None	Cream	Saline	Paste
4.5- 4.5	116[†]	104	103	93
8.0- 8.0	90	66	71	64
8.0-12.8	80	60	60	54
12.8-12.8	57	49	50	45

*From Connell, P. N., Ewy, G. A., Dahl, C. F., and Ewy, M. D.: Transthoracic resistance to defibrillator discharge: effect of electrode–chest wall interface. In preparation.
[†]Mean values in ohms.

Table 3. Myocardial damage produced by ten consecutive DC defibrillator discharges at a dial setting of 400 watt-seconds*

Time interval between discharges	Paddle electrode size[†]		
	4.5 cm.	8.0 cm.	12.8 cm.
15 seconds		+++	++
1 minute		++	
3 minutes	++	+	

*From Dahl, C. F., Ewy, G. A., Warner, E. D., and Ewy, M. D.: Myocardial damage from direct current defibrillator discharge. In preparation.
[†]+, Relative damage estimated by degree of S-T segment elevation present on precordial mapping.

Adverse effects

The erythematous haloes on a patient's chest following defibrillation or cardioversion are a familiar sight; although they are sometimes painful to the patient, they are not regarded as serious by most physicians. Enzymes such as CPK and SGOT have been measured following cardioversion; while they were found to be increased, most reports concluded that such elevations were the result of damage to chest wall muscle rather than to cardiac tissue.[6,7]

During our studies on canine transthoracic resistance, however, we noted myocardial damage aften ten countershocks. To see whether damage could be reduced, we tried the following experiment. Ten discharges of equal energy level were delivered to five groups of animals, the variables being *time* between countershocks and *paddle size* used to deliver the shocks. The results are summarized in Table 3. It can be seen that damage was greatest when small paddles were used and shocks delivered at frequent intervals. Damage could be decreased by using larger size paddles and by waiting longer intervals between delivery of shocks.[8]

These problems were brought into focus recently when a salesman showed me the latest model of a defibrillator (Statham Model SM-1210) and pointed out that it actually delivered the energy indicated on the dial. Evaluation of the device revealed that it did indeed deliver close to 100, 200, 300, and 400 watt-seconds of energy into a 50-ohm resistive load at the respective dial settings. When the dial was set on "max" it delivered 580 watt-seconds. This increased capacity for delivering

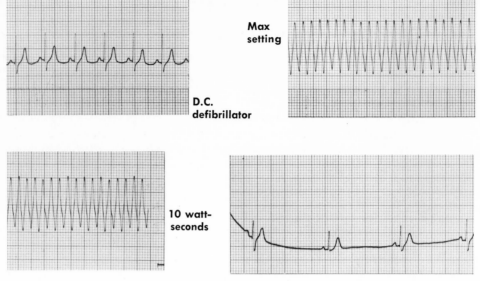

**Max
setting**

**D.C.
defibrillator**

**10 watt-
seconds**

Dog 72-0

Fig. 21-3. Electrocardiogram of dog given one discharge at Max setting (see text) from a direct current discharge. Top left: Sinus rhythm. Top right: Ventricular flutter. Bottom left: Ventricular flutter. Bottom right: Sinus bradycardia that persisted only a short time after cardioversion with an additional 10 watt-seconds.

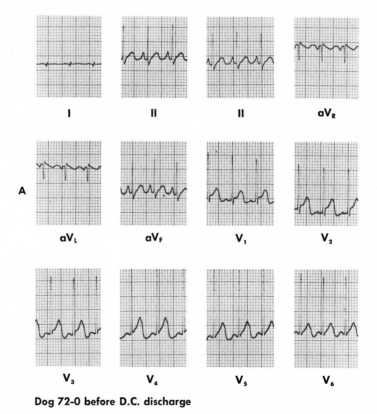

I   II   II   aV$_R$

A   aV$_L$ aV$_F$ V$_1$ V$_2$

V$_3$ V$_4$ V$_5$ V$_6$

Dog 72-0 before D.C. discharge

Fig. 21-4. Standard twelve-lead electrocardiograms on a dog before **(A)** and after **(B)** one maximal direct current discharge via pediatric paddle electrodes (see text).

energy may be very helpful in certain large patients. However, this particular device had pediatric-size paddles with paddle electrodes that measured 4.5 cm in diameter. Having just completed the studies referred to in Tables 2 and 3, I was concerned about such a unit as this (or units with similar capacity) being used on the pediatric wards. In an emergency situation the dial could be turned fully clockwise to the "max" setting. In all probability, a considerable amount of myocardial damage would result from delivery of 580 watt-seconds of energy when using a pediatric paddle.

To test this hypothesis, the machine was taken to our animal laboratory. As illustrated in Fig. 21-3, one shock delivered at maximal setting resulted in rapid ventricular flutter. A 10 watt-second discharge was delivered to break the flutter. Fig. 21-4 shows a twelve-lead electrocardiogram taken after the discharge, which revealed multiple premature ventricular contractions as well as S-T segment elevations across the precordial leads. This experience dramatically reinforced the importance of being fully aware of the performance characteristics of the defibrillator one is planning to use, either in an emergency or in an elective situation. Only in this way can one hope to arrive at an electric prescription that is both safe and effective.

Although research continues, certain guidelines for defibrillation or cardioversion can be set forth at this time.

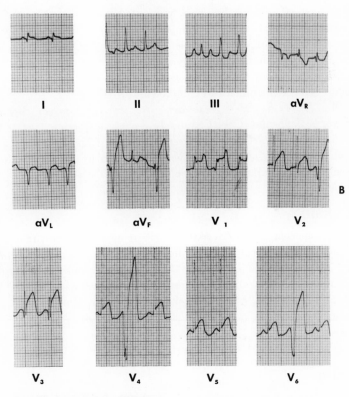

Dog 72-0 after D.C. discharge

Fig. 21-4, cont'd. For legend see opposite page.

DEFIBRILLATION GUIDELINES

1. *Deliver the defibrillatory countershock as soon as possible.* Cardiopulmonary resuscitation (CPR) is barely adequate and is not sufficient to sustain life in the majority of instances. If it were, there would be many patients stricken some distance from the hospital who would be sustained by CPR until they could be brought to the hospital for defibrillation and who would thus survive. This does not occur.[9] Therefore, mobile coronary care units are being developed in which the defibrillator is taken to the patient. The ineffectiveness of external cardiac massage over a long period of time is not surprising. Cardiac contraction is a complicated process that requires the active participation of the papillary muscles to close the mitral valve so that blood can be ejected into the aorta. When the heart is passively compressed between the sternum and the vertebral column, gross mitral regurgitation results and cardiac output is not sufficient to sustain life more than a few minutes.

2. *Use large paddles with saline-soaked gauze pads or electrode paste as the electrode–chest wall interface.* Resistance is decreased with increased paddle size; therefore, more current is delivered from a fixed energy level discharge. In an emergency situation, many operators like to use saline-soaked gauze pads so that CPR can be continued uninterruptedly between countershocks without having a slippery chest for compression. This is an acceptable compromise. However, in large patients where optimal resistance-lowering is desired, electrode *paste* may be more effective.

3. *Deliver two or three shocks in rapid succession when one maximal countershock does not produce the desired result.* The rationale for this has been difficult to understand, since it has been postulated that all of the myofibrils had to be depolarized to effect defibrillation. A recent report from investigators using internal wire electrodes for ventricular defibrillation has shown that one shock of an energy level inadequate for defibrillation made the fibrillatory waves coarse; a second, subdefibrillatory shock made them coarser; and a third or fourth shock of the same energy level resulted in a reversion to sinus rhythm.[10]

4. *It may be necessary to administer drugs before you conclude that the patient cannot be defibrillated.* See Chapter 16.

5. *Once defibrillation has been successful, attempt to determine the factors precipitating fibrillation.* We have been impressed by the number of times drugs such as digitalis or quinidine have contributed to the development of ventricular fibrillation.

CARDIOVERSION

The concept of cardioversion is based on the premise that the sustaining mechanism of atrial fibrillation is different from the initiating mechanism.[11,12] Thus, if the initiating mechanism is no longer present and the sustaining mechanism is terminated, sinus rhythm will ensue. In many instances the initiating mechanism—severe heart failure, mitral stenosis, a giant left atrium, a recent pulmonary embolus, pneumonia, and so on—is still present; therefore, attempting cardioversion is not advisable.

The indications for cardioversion are outlined in Chapter 9.

Premedications

I prefer to give the patient anticoagulants for 2 weeks prior to cardioversion and for 6 months afterward. This preference is based on the clinical study performed by

Bjerkelund and Orning,[13] in which they found that emboli occurred in eleven of 209 patients not receiving anticoagulation and in only two of 228 patients receiving anticoagulation. Emboli occurred as long as 6 months after cardioversion.

If there are no contraindications, administer quinidine sulfate in 200-mg doses, four times a day, at least 2 days before and doses of 300 mg, four times a day, in the 24 hours preceding cardioversion. The purpose of giving quinidine prior to cardioversion is threefold[14]:

1. To see whether the patient can tolerate a maintenance dose of quinidine
2. To see whether the patient will revert to sinus rhythm on quinidine alone
3. To use less energy to successfully electrically cardiovert patients on maintenance quinidine

Some patients will revert to sinus rhythm with small doses of quinidine and thus can be spared the discomfort of cardioversion. Higher doses of quinidine, which produce blood levels between 5 and 7 mg/liter, pose risk of serious arrhythmias at the time of cardioversion.[15]

If diazepam (Valium) is used for sedation, two aspects are worthy of emphasis. First, the drug should be administered directly into the vein and not into intravenous tubing, since it will precipitate in saline or glucose and water solutions. Second, some patients require a high dosage for sedation; this usually is the case in patients who have been taking high doses of tranquilizers and/or sedatives. In such a situation we usually give no more than 30 mg; if the patient still is not adequately sedated, morphine sulfate will be administered and the countershock delivered. Those not familiar with diazepam should have a qualified anesthesiologist administer it or another appropriate anesthetic.

Make sure the patient does not have digitalis excess. The diagnosis of digitalis excess is more difficult in the presence of atrial fibrillation.[16] Attention should be paid to slow ventricular response rate, regularization of ventricular response, group beating, and/or premature ventricular contractions (see Chapter 12). If any of these phenomena are present, cardioversion should be delayed. Some advise stopping digoxin 48 hours and digitoxin 72 hours before cardioversion. This is not necessary if there is no evidence of digitalis excess. If there is any question, digitalis should be discontinued and the procedure delayed.

Technique

Cardioversion should be carried out in a well-equipped coronary care unit so that pre- or postconversion arrhythmias can be noted quickly by an alert and well-trained nursing staff and any complications treated quickly and efficiently.

1. *Patient should have been fasting for 12 hours prior to cardioversion, except for quinidine therapy.*
2. *Have intravenous lidocaine on hand.*
3. *Make sure cardioverter is properly synchronized.*
4. *Use large, anterior-posterior paddle electrode placement.* Dr. Lown has shown that it takes less energy to cardiovert patients when anterior-posterior paddles are used in contrast to anterior-lateral paddles.[17]
5. *Use gritty electrode paste.* Our studies have shown that the resistance to a direct current shock is decreased by using electrode *paste* rather than saline-soaked gauze pads or electrode cream.[5]
6. *Deliver small energy discharge and observe electrocardiogram for repetitive*

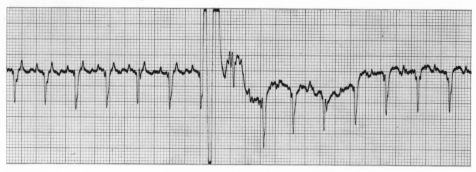

3 watt-second setting

Fig. 21-5. Electrocardiogram illustrating low energy test discharge in a patient with atrial flutter. No repetitive firing was seen. The patient was cardioverted with a subsequent 10 watt-second discharge.

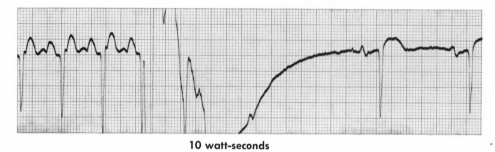

10 watt-seconds

Fig. 21-6. Electrocardiogram illustrating cardioversion of atrial flutter with 10 watt-second discharge via anterior-posterior paddle electrodes using electrode paste as interface.

firing. This has been recommended by Dr. Lown. Fig. 21-5 illustrates one such test discharge in a patient with flutter that did not result in repetitive firing. The next discharge of 10 watt-seconds cardioverted the patient. Low energy cardioversion occurs most frequently in flutter, as shown in Fig. 21-6, in which a flutter was converted with a 10 watt-second discharge.

7. *Do not rely on monitor leads alone to determine if sinus rhythm has been restored.* Take a standard twelve-lead electrocardiogram.

8. *Wait at least 3 minutes between discharges.* I have often seen cardioversions performed in which the patient was sedated or anesthetized and discharges of 50, 100, 200, 300, and 400 watt-seconds were delivered in rapid sequence before the sedation wore off. The potential risk of chest wall and cardiac damage can be decreased by spacing discharges at appropriate time intervals (see Table 3).

9. *Change cardioverter to defibrillator as soon as the shock is delivered and palpate femoral or carotid pulse.* If the patient develops ventricular fibrillation and one attempts to defibrillate with the cardioverter, nothing will happen, since the latter device is programmed to discharge on the spike of the R wave. With ventricular fibrillation, there is no distinct R wave.

10. *Observe the patient after cardioversion.* Watch the patient for signs of development of serious arrhythmias or potentially serious rhythms, such as sick sinus syndrome.

REFERENCES

1. Ewy, G. A., Fletcher, R. D., and Ewy, M. D.: Comparative analysis of direct current defibrillators, J. Electrocardiol. **5**:349, 1972.
2. Geddes, L., Tacker, W., Rosborough, J., and Cabler, P.: Trans-chest defibrillation of heavy subjects (abstract), Circulation **46**:II-108, 1972.
3. Sutton, W. A., Galysh, F. T., and Hagan, W. K.: Significant determinants of successful reversion of fibrillation by a new DC defibrillator: an experimental study, Am. Heart J. **79**:630-639, 1970.
4. Patel, A. S., and Galysh, F. T.: Experimental studies to design safe external pediatric paddles for a DC defibrillator, I.E.E.E. Trans. Bio-Med. Eng. **BME-19**:228, 1972.
5. Connell, P. N., Ewy, G. A., Dahl, C. F., and Ewy, M. D.: Transthoracic resistance to defibrillator discharge: effect of electrode-chest wall interface. In preparation.
6. Konttinen, A., Hupli, V., Louhija, A., and Hartel, G.: Origin of elevated serum enzyme activities after direct-current countershock, New Eng. J. Med. **281**:231, 1969.
7. Mandecki, T., Giec, L., and Kargul, W.: Serum enzyme activities after cardioversion, Brit. Heart J. **32**:600, 1970.
8. Dahl, C. F., Ewy, G. A., Warner, E. D., and Ewy, M. D.: Myocardial damage from direct current defibrillator discharge. In preparation.
9. Wilder, R. J., Jude, J. R., Kouwenhoven, W. B., and McMahon, M. C.: Cardiopulmonary resuscitations by trained ambulance personnel, J.A.M.A. **190**:531, 1964.
10. Mower, M. M., Mirowski, M., and Moore, E. N.: Patterns of intraventricular catheter defibrillation (abstract), Circulation **46**:II-25, 1972.
11. Lown, B., Amarasingham, R., and Neuman, J.: New method for terminating cardiac arrhythmias: use of synchronized capacitor discharge, J.A.M.A. **182**:548, 1962.
12. Lown, B.: Electrical reversion of cardiac arrhythmias, Brit. Heart J. **29**:469-489, 1967.
13. Bjerkelund, C. J., and Orning, O. M.: The efficacy of anticoagulant therapy in preventing embolism related to D.C. electrical conversion of atrial fibrillation, Am. J. Cardiol. **23**:208-216, 1969
14. Rossi, M., and Lown, B.: The use of quinidine in cardioversion, Am. J. Cardiol. **19**:234-238, 1967.
15. Aberg, H., and Cullhed, I.: Direct current countershock complications, Acta Med. Scand. **183**:415-421, 1968.
16. Kastor, J. A., and Yurchak, P. M.: Recognition of digitalis intoxication in the presence of atrial fibrillation, Ann. Intern. Med. **67**:1045, 1967.
17. Lown, B., Kleiger, R., and Wolff, G.: The technique of cardioversion, Am. Heart J. **67**:282, 1964.

INDEX

A

Aberrant conduction
  intraventricular, versus ventricular ectopic firing,
    161-162
  Marriott's criteria for, 162
Aberration, ventricular, 44-46
Alcoholic myocardiopathy, atrial fibrillation in, car-
    dioversion for, 88
Anatomy of conducting tissues of heart, 3, 4
Anticoagulant therapy, chronic, for chronic atrial fi-
    brillation, 90
Arrhythmias
  complex, 111-176
    accelerated ectopic rhythm with atrioventricular
      block, 144-145
    chaotic rhythms, 147, 148
    concealed conduction into atrioventricular node,
      145-146
    digitalis-induced, 113-127
    fatal, 150-154
    high degree of atrioventricular block with inter-
      fering atrioventricular junctional rhythm,
      142-144
    idioatrial rhythm, 158, 159
    interference-dissociation combined with atrio-
      ventricular block, 142, 143
    rate-dependent bundle branch block, 146-148
    sick sinus syndrome, 135-141
    wandering pacemaker, 158, 159
  in coronary care unit, 150-154
  digitalis-induced; see Digitalis, arrhythmias in-
    duced by
  fatal, 150-154
    treatment, 152-154
    ventricular fibrillation, 150, 151
    ventricular flutter, 150-152
    ventricular standstill, 152
  simple, 11-110
    atrial fibrillation, 82-90
    atrial flutter, 91-97
    atrioventricular block, 59-81
    ectopic beats, 16-28
    sustained ectopic rhythms, 29-43
    ventricular aberration, 44-46
    ventricular fusion, 46-49
  sinus, 14-15

Arteries, coronary, disease of, as cause of atrial fi-
    brillation, 82
Ashman phenomenon, 161-162
Atrial ectopic beats; see Ectopic beats, atrial
Atrial fibrillation; see Fibrillation, atrial
Atrial flutter; see Flutter, atrial
Atrial pacing, 187
  for atrioventricular junctional or ventricular
    rhythms, 155
  for escape ectopic rhythms, 42
  for interference-dissociation
    due to paroxysmal tachycardia, 134
    due to slowing of sinoatrial node, 134
  for severe sinus bradycardia, 155
Atrial rhythm, chaotic, 147, 148
Atrial syncytium, anatomy, 3
Atrial tachycardia, 31-33
  multifocal, 135
Atrioventricular (A-V) block, 59-81
  accelerated ectopic rhythm with, 144-145
  anatomic site, 59-60
  bifascicular, 75, 76, 77
  classification, 59
    functional, 60-78
  clinical diagnosis, 79
  complete, 69, 70-71
    analysis, 101-102, 167-168
    with atrial flutter or fibrillation, 120, 121
    definition, 130
    treatment, 80
  fascicular, in bundle branch system, 73, 75
    analysis, 109
  first-degree, 60-62
    treatment, 79
  high degree, with interfering atrioventricular junc-
    tional rhythm, 142-144
  interference-dissociation combined with, 142, 143
  localized in bundle branches, 71-73, 74
  myocardial infarction with, insertion of pacing
    catheter for, 156
  paroxysmal atrial tachycardia with, caused by digi-
    talis toxicity, 115-120
  second-degree, 62-69
    with fixed ratio/fixed P-R interval, 62, 63, 64
    Mobitz Type 2, 68-69
      analysis, 99-100, 169

198

Atrioventricular (A-V) block—cont'd
  second-degree—cont'd
    treatment, 79
      with Wenckebach phenomenon, 62, 64-68; *see also* Wenckebach phenomenon
    severe, analysis, 107-108
    symptoms, 78
    treatment, 79-80
    trifascicular, 75-76
Atrioventricular (A-V) bundle, anatomy, 3
Atrioventricular (A-V) dissociation, 128
Atrioventricular (A-V) junctional beats, 23-25
Atrioventricular (A-V) junctional tachycardia, 31
Atrioventricular (A-V) node
  anatomy, 3
  concealed conduction into, 145-146
Atropine, 183-184
  administration, in detection of sick sinus syndrome, 140
  for atrioventricular junctional or ventricular rhythms, 155
  for digitalis-induced atrioventricular block or sinoatrial node depression, 126
  for escape ectopic rhythms
    due to failure of conduction from atria to ventricles, 41
    due to inadequate rate of discharge of sinoatrial node, 41
  for interference-dissociation
    due to paroxysmal tachycardia, 134
    due to slowing of sinoatrial node, 134
  for severe sinus bradycardia, 155
  in treatment of atrioventricular block, 80
A-V node; *see* Atrioventricular (A-V) node

B

Beats
  capture, 132-133
  ectopic; *see* Ectopic beats
Belladonna, tincture of, 183-184
Beta-adrenergic blocking agents, 183
  for supraventricular tachycardias associated with pre-excitation, 161
Bifascicular block, 75, 76, 77
Bigeminal rhythm
  atrioventricular, 24-25
  ventricular, 26
    with atrial fibrillation, analysis, 167-168
Bradycardia, sinus, 14, 136
  analysis, 57-58
  as cause of interference-dissociation, 130, 131
  due to digitalis toxicity, 123
  persistent, 135
  severe, treatment, 155-156
Bradycardia-tachycardia syndrome, 138-140
Bretylium tosylate, 183
Bundle of His, anatomy, 3
Bundle branches
  atrioventricular block localized in, 71-73, 74
    fascicular, 73, 75
  block of, 44-45
    analysis, 106-107
    atrioventricular junctional beats with, 55-56
    left, 174-175
    rate-dependent, 146-148

Bundle branches—cont'd
  block of—cont'd
    right and left, 56-57
      distinguishing between, 45, 46
    and ventricular ectopic beats, differentiation between, 45

C

Calcium chloride for ventricular standstill, 153
Capture, 130
Capture beats, 132-133
  analysis, 170-172
  in interference-dissociation with atrioventricular block, 142, 143
Cardiac; *see* Heart
Cardioversion, 194-196
  of atrial fibrillation, 87-89
    excessive risk with, 88
    quinidine for, 89
    sick sinus syndrome following, 139, 140
  of atrial flutter, 96-97
  premedications, 194-195
  for supraventricular tachycardia, 36
  technique, 195-196
Carotid sinus, stimulation of, in diagnosis of sick sinus syndrome, 140-141
Catheter, pacing, insertion of, in myocardial infarction with atrioventricular block, 156
Chaotic rhythms
  atrial, 147, 148
    analysis, 170
  ventricular, 148
Compensatory pause in ectopic beats, 27-28
Complex arrhythmias; *see* Arrhythmias, complex
Conducting tissues of heart
  anatomy, 3
  nervous control, 6
  refractory period, 6-7
Conduction
  aberrant
    intraventricular, versus ventricular ectopic firing, 161-162
    Marriott's criteria for, 162
  from atria to ventricles, escape ectopic rhythms due to failure of, treatment, 41-42
  into atrioventricular node, concealed, 145-146
Coronary care unit
  arrhythmias in, 150-154
  equipment for, 155

D

Defibrillation
  guidelines for, 194
  for ventricular fibrillation, 152
Defibrillators, 188-191
  adverse effects, 191-193
Deslanoside for supraventricular tachycardia, 36
Diagnosis
  of atrial fibrillation, 84-87
  of atrial flutter, 91-96
  bedside, of ectopic beats, 27
  clinical, of atrioventricular block, 79
  electrocardiographic; *see* Electrocardiographic diagnosis
  of sick sinus syndrome, steps in, 140-141

Diazepam as premedication for cardioversion, 195
Digitalis, 179-180; *see also* Digitalization
  arrhythmias induced by, 113-127
    analysis, 172
    bidirectional paroxysmal ventricular tachycardia, 123
    clinical considerations and correlations, 123-124
    complete atrioventricular block, analysis, 167-168
    complex arrhythmias caused by digitalis toxicity, 114-122
    delay or block of premature atrial beats, 114-115, 116
    depression of sinus node function, 122-123
    ectopic nodal and ventricular discharge interrupting atrial flutter and fibrillation, 120, 121-122
    junctional tachycardia, analysis, 168-169
    paroxysmal atrial tachycardia with atrioventricular block, 115-120
      analysis, 164-165, 175
    treatment, 125-126
  for escape ectopic rhythms due to failure of conduction from atria to ventricles, 41
  for slowing of ventricular rate in atrial fibrillation, 85, 86, 89-90
  for supraventricular tachycardia, 35-36
  in treatment of sick sinus syndrome, 141
Digitalis leaf, 180
Digitalization
  for atrial flutter, 96
  modes, 90
  slow, 179
Digitoxin, 180
Digoxin, 179-180
  for digitalization for atrial fibrillation, 90
  for supraventricular tachycardia, 35-36
Dilantin; *see* Diphenylhydantoin
Diphenylhydantoin, 182
  for digitalis-induced ventricular tachyarrhythmias, 125-126
  for supraventricular tachycardia, 36
Dissociation
  atrioventricular, 128
  isorhythmic, 133
Dressler beat, 48
Drugs
  atropine, 183-184
  beta-adrenergic blocking agents, 183
  bretylium tosylate, 183
  deslanoside, 180
  digitalis, 179-180
  digitalis leaf, 180
  digitoxin, 180
  Dilantin, 182
  diphenylhydantoin, 182
  and dosages, 179-184
  edrophonium, 182-183
  lidocaine, 182
  procainamide, 181
  Pronestyl, 181
  quinidine, 180-181
  for supraventricular tachycardia
    sympathomimetic, 35
    vagomimetic, 35

Drugs—cont'd
  Tensilon, 182-183
  for ventricular fibrillation, 152-153
  for ventricular standstill, 153

E

Ectopic beats, 16-28
  atrial, 21, 25
    atrioventricular nodal (junctional), 23-25
    escape, 22-23
    premature, 21-22
  clinical aspects, 27-28
  escape; *see* Escape ectopic beats
  origin, recognizing site of, 19-27
  parasystolic focus, 162-163
  premature; *see* Premature ectopic beats
  ventricular, 25-27
    aberrant intraventricular conduction versus, 161-162
    and bundle branch block, differentiation between, 45
    interrupting atrial fibrillation, 102
    interrupting paroxysmal atrial flutter, 102-104
    lidocaine for, 182
    in production of ventricular fibrillation, 150
    quinidine for, 181
Ectopic pacemakers, mechanism of action, 16-18
Ectopic rhythms
  accelerated, with atrioventricular block, 144-145
  active, 29
  escape, 29; *see also* Escape ectopic rhythms
  sustained, 29-43
    escape or passive, 38-42
    paroxysmal tachycardia; *see* Paroxysmal tachycardia
Edrophonium, 182-183
  for supraventricular tachycardia, 35
Electrocardiogram
  normal, 13, 14
  time measurements in, 8-10
  waves; *see* Waves of electrocardiogram
Electrocardiographic diagnosis
  of atrial and atrioventricular junctional tachycardia, 31-33
  of atrial fibrillation, 85-87
  of atrial flutter, 93-96
  of sinus rhythms, 13
  of Wenckebach phenomenon, 67
Electroshock; *see* Electroversion
Electroversion
  of atrial flutter, 96
  for converting atrial fibrillation to sinus rhythm, 87-88
  for supraventricular tachycardia, 36
  for ventricular tachycardia, 38
Emboli, danger of, in chronic atrial fibrillation, 84
Endotracheal intubation during cardiac arrest, rules governing, 156-157
Epinephrine
  for ventricular fibrillation, 152-153
  for ventricular standstill, 153
Escape ectopic beats
  atrial, 22, 23
  mechanism of action, 16-18
  ventricular, 27

Escape ectopic pacemakers, mechanism of action, 16-18
Escape ectopic rhythms, 38-42
  idionodal and idioventricular, relation to cardiac output, 42
  as symptom of digitalis toxicity, 113-114
  treatment, 41-42
Escape interference, 130-132

F

Fascicular block in the bundle branch system, 73, 75
Fatal arrhythmias; *see* Arrhythmias, fatal
Fibers, Purkinje, anatomy, 3
Fibrillation
  atrial, 82-90
    analysis, 98, 99, 100-101
    atrioventricular junctional rhythm interrupting, analysis, 104-105
    cardioversion of, 87-89
      sick sinus syndrome following, 139, 140
    causes, 82
    complete atrioventricular block with, 120, 121
    conversion to sinus rhythm, 87-89
    diagnosis, 84-87
    flutter-fibrillation, 86, 87
    junctional or ventricular paroxysmal tachycardia with, 121-122
    lone, cardioversion for, 88
    mechanism, 82, 83
    premature ventricular beats interrupting, 120, 121
    quinidine for, 180-181
    significance, 84
    treatment, 87-90
    with ventricular bigeminy, analysis, 167-168
  ventricular ectopic beats interrupting, analysis, 102
  ventricular, 150, 151
    treatment, 152-153
First-degree atrioventricular block, 60-62
Flutter
  atrial, 91-97
    analysis, 99, 106-107
    cardioversion, 96-97
    clinical manifestations, 96
    complete atrioventricular block with, 120, 121
    diagnosis, 91-96
    edrophonium for diagnosis, 182
    mechanism, 91, 92
    paroxysmal, with ventricular ectopic firing, analysis, 102-104
    premature ventricular beats interrupting, 120, 121
    quinidine for, 180-181
    treatment, 96-97
  ventricular, 150-152
Flutter-fibrillation, 86, 87
Fusion, ventricular, 46-49
Fusion beats, 48-49
  analysis, 50, 51
  in atrial fibrillation interrupted by ventricular ectopic beats, 102
  significance, 49

H

Heart
  complete block, 69, 70-71
    analysis, 101-102
  conducting tissues
    anatomy and physiology, 3-7
    schematic representation, 4
  disease
    congenital, as cause of atrial fibrillation, 82
    hypertensive, atrial fibrillation in, cardioversion for, 88
    rheumatic, as cause of atrial fibrillation, 82
  output, relation to idionodal and idioventricular rhythms, 42
  pacemaker; *see* Pacemaker(s)
  resuscitation, 156-157
Heartbeat, normal, physiology, 3-7
His, bundle of, anatomy, 3
Holter monitor recording for diagnosing sick sinus syndrome, 140, 141
Hypoxemia, chronic atrial, enhancement of digitalis toxicity by, 124

I

Idioatrial rhythms, 29, 158, 159; *see also* Escape ectopic rhythms
Idionodal rhythms; 29; *see also* Escape ectopic rhythms
Idioventricular rhythms, 29; *see also* Escape ectopic rhythms
  analysis, 52, 53
  during atrial fibrillation, 86, 87
Inderal for supraventricular tachycardia, 36
Interference
  analysis, 57-58
  definition, 128-130
  escape, 130-132
Interference-dissociation
  analysis, 170-172
  clinical significance and treatment, 133-134
  combined with atrioventricular block, 142, 143
  mechanisms, 130-132
Intubation, endotracheal, during cardiac arrest, rules governing, 156-157
Isoproterenol
  for atrioventricular block, 80
  for digitalis-induced arrhythmias, dangers in, 126
  for escape ectopic rhythms
    due to failure of conduction from atria to ventricles, 41
    due to inadequate rate of discharge of sinoatrial node, 41
Isorhythmic dissociation, 133

K

Kidneys, impaired function, enhancement of digitalis toxicity by, 124

L

Lanatoside C for digitalization for atrial fibrillation, 90
Lanoxin; *see* Digoxin
Lead V in distinguishing left and right bundle branch block, 45, 46

Lidocaine, 182
    for digitalis-induced ventricular tachyarrhythmias, 126
    for ventricular tachycardia, 36-37
Lown-Ganong-Levine syndrome, 161

M

Marriott's criteria of aberrancy versus ectopy, 162
Massage, open chest, in treatment of ventricular standstill, 153-154
Mitral valve stenosis as cause of atrial fibrillation, 82
Mobitz Type 2 atrioventricular block, 68-69
    localized in bundle branches, 73, 74
Mural thrombi in chronic atrial fibrillation, 84
Myocardial infarction with atrioventricular block, insertion of pacing catheter for, 156
Myocardiopathy, alcoholic, atrial fibrillation in, cardioversion, for, 88

N

Neostigmine for supraventricular tachycardia, 35
Neo-Synephrine for supraventricular tachycardia, 35
Nerve fibers
    parasympathetic, inhibitory effects on conducting system, 6
    sympathetic, cardioaccelerary effects on conducting system, 6
    vagal, indirect effects on conducting system, 6
Nerves in control of conducting system, 6
Nodes
    atrioventricular (A-V), anatomy, 3
    sinoatrial (S-A), anatomy, 3

O

Open chest massage for ventricular standstill, 153-154
Ouabain for digitalization for atrial fibrillation, 90

P

P waves
    absence, in diagnosis of atrial fibrillation, 85
    in accelerated ectopic rhythm with atrioventricular block, 144-145
    in atrial escape ectopic beats, 22-23
    in atrioventricular block
        complete, 69, 70-71
        with interfering atrioventricular junctional rhythm, 142-144
        second-degree
            with fixed P-R interval, 62, 63, 64
            Mobitz Type 2, 68-69
                localized in bundle branch, 74
            Wenckebach phenomenon, 62, 64-68
    in bradycardia-tachycardia syndromes, 138-140
    in chaotic rhythms, 147, 148
    in concealed conduction into atrioventricular node, 145-146
    in diagnosis of arrhythmias, 4-5
    in differentiation of atrial and atrioventricular junctional tachycardia, 31-32
    in differentiation between ventricular ectopic beats and bundle branch block, 45
    in digitalis-induced paroxysmal atrial tachycardia with atrioventricular block, 117, 118, 120
    in escape ectopic rhythms, 38-41

P waves—cont'd
    in idioatrial rhythm, 158, 159
    in interference-dissociation caused by escape junctional rhythm in sinus bradycardia, 131
    in isorhythmic dissociation, 133
    in normal sinus rhythm, 13
    in premature atrial beats, 21-22
        blocked or delayed by digitalis toxicity, 115, 116
    in prolonged postectopic pauses in sick sinus syndrome, 136
    relation to QRS in atrioventricular junctional beats, 23-25
    relation to ventricular complex, 20
    retrograde, in diagnosing of ventricular tachycardia, 33-34
    significance of, 4-5
    in sinoatrial block in sick sinus syndrome, 136-138
    in ventricular ectopic beats, 25-27
Pacemaker(s)
    ectopic
        atrial, functions, 23
        mechanism of action, 16-17
    permanent, in treatment of atrioventricular block, 80
    sinoatrial node as, 3-4
    temporary transvenous
        insertion of, 185-187
        in treatment of atrioventricular block, 80
    wandering, 158, 159
Pacers and pacing, 185-187
Pacing
    atrial, 187
        for atrioventricular junctional or ventricular rhythms, 155
        for escape ectopic rhythms, 42
        for interference-dissociation
            due to paroxysmal tachycardia, 134
            due to slowing of sinoatrial node, 134
        for severe sinus bradycardia, 155
    permanent, indications for, 185
    temporary, indications for, 185
    ventricular, 187
        for digitalis-induced atrioventricular block or sinoatrial node depression, 126
        for sick sinus syndrome, 141
        for ventricular standstill, 153
Pacing catheter, insertion of, in myocardial infarction with atrioventricular block, 156
Parasympathetic nerve fibers, effects on conducting system, 6
Parasystole, 162-163
Paroxysmal tachycardia, 29-38
    atrial
        with atrioventricular block caused by digitalis toxicity, 115-120
        analysis, 164-165, 175
        and atrioventricular junctional, 31-33
    as cause of interference-dissociation, 132
    clinical manifestations, 34
    junctional or ventricular, with atrial fibrillation, 121-122
    supraventricular, 31-33
        analysis, 53
        therapy, 35-36
    as symptom of digitalis toxicity, 113

Paroxysmal tachycardia—cont'd
  therapy, 34-38
  vagal stimulation, 34
  ventricular, 33-34
    analysis, 52, 54
    bidirectional, 123
    therapy, 36-38
Phenylephrine hydrochloride for supraventricular
    tachycardia, 35
Physiology
  of conducting tissues of heart, 3-7
  of normal heartbeat, 3-7
Postectopic pauses, 27-28
  prolonged, in sick sinus syndrome, 136
Postmature ectopic beats; *see* Escape ectopic beats
Potassium
  for digitalis-induced arrhythmias with potassium
    depletion, 125
  for digitalis-induced paroxysmal atrial tachycardia
    with atrioventricular block, 117
  elevated, for escape ectopic rhythms due to failure
    of conduction from atria to ventricles, 41
  low serum levels, enhancement of digitalis toxicity
    by, 124
P-R interval, 8, 9
  in Ashman phenomenon, 161-162
  in atrioventricular block
    complete, 69, 70-71
    first-degree, 60-62
      in adults, 60-62
      in children, 62
      localized in bundle branches, 72
    second-degree
      with fixed P-R, 62, 63, 64
      localized in bundle branches, 73, 74
      Mobitz Type 2, 68-69
        localized in bundle branch, 74
      Wenckebach phenomenon, 62, 64-68
  in capture beat in analysis of condition of atrio-
    ventricular conducting tissues, 133
  in concealed conduction into atrioventricular node,
    145-146
  in digitalis-induced paroxysmal atrial tachycardia
    with atrioventricular block, 116, 118
  in interference-dissociation with atrioventricular
    block, 142, 143
  prolonged
    in premature atrial beats as indication of digi-
      talis toxicity, 114-115, 116
    as symptom of digitalis toxicity, 113
  short, in diagnosis of pre-excitation, 160
  in Wolff-Parkinson-White syndrome, 158-160
Practolol, 183
Pre-excitation (Wolff-Parkinson-White syndrome),
    158-161
Premature ectopic beats
  atrial, 21-22
    analysis, 53-54
    delay or block of, due to digitalis toxicity, 114-
      115, 116
  atrioventricular junctional, analysis, 57-58
  mechanism of action, 16-17
  as symptom of digitalis toxicity, 113
  ventricular, 26
    atrial fibrillation interrupted by, 86, 120, 121

Premature ectopic pacemakers, mechanism of action,
    16-18
Procainamide, 181
  for digitalis-induced ventricular tachyarrhythmias,
    126
  for supraventricular tachycardia, 36
  for ventricular tachycardia, 37
Pronestyl, 181
  for ventricular tachycardia, 37
Propranolol, 183
  for supraventricular tachycardia, 36
Prostigmin for supraventricular tachycardia, 35
Pulse deficit in diagnosis of atrial fibrillation, 84
Pulsus bigeminus, analysis, 54-55
Purkinje fibers, anatomy, 3
PVC; *see* Premature ectopic beats, ventricular

Q

QRS complex; *see* Ventricular (QRS) complex
QRS interval, 8, 9
Quinidine, 180-181
  for cardioversion
    for atrial fibrillation, 89
    for atrial flutter, 96-97
  for digitalis-induced arrhythmias, dangers in, 126
  for escape ectopic rhythms due to failure of con-
    duction from atria to ventricles, 41
  in maintenance of sinus rhythm, 89
  as premedication for cardioversion, 195
  for supraventricular tachycardia, 36
  for ventricular tachycardia, 37-38

R

Rate-dependent bundle branch block, 146-148
Refractory period of conducting tissues, 6-7
Renal function, impaired, enhancement of digitalis
    toxicity by, 124
Resuscitation, cardiac, 156-157
Rhythms
  atrioventricular junctional
    analysis, 172-174
    treatment, 155
    or ventricular, accelerated, as cause of interfer-
      ence-dissociation, 130, 131
  chaotic
    atrial, 147, 148
    ventricular, 148
  ectopic; *see* Ectopic rhythms
  idioatrial, 29, 158, 159; *see also* Escape ectopic
    rhythms
  idionodal, 29; *see also* Escape ectopic rhythms
  idioventricular, 29; *see also* Escape ectopic rhythms
    analysis, 52-53
    during atrial fibrillation, 86, 87
  sinus, 13-15; *see also* Sinus rhythms
  ventricular, treatment, 155

S

S-A node; *see* Sinoatrial (S-A) node
Second-degree atrioventricular block, 62-69
Sick sinus syndrome, 135-141
  with bradycardia-tachycardia, 138-140
  following cardioversion of atrial fibrillation, 139,
    140
  clinical manifestations, 135-136

Sick sinus syndrome—cont'd
diagnosis of, steps in, 140-141
as indication for temporary and permanent pacing, 185
with prolonged postectopic pause, 136
with sinoatrial block, 136-138
with sinus bradycardia, 136
treatment, 141
types of, 136-140
as warning of digitalis toxicity, 123
Simple arrhythmias; *see* Arrhythmias, simple
Sinoatrial (S-A) block, 136-138
Sinoatrial (S-A) node
anatomy, 3
function, digitalis depression of, 122-123
inadequate rate of discharge, escape ectopic rhythms due to, treatment, 41
overdrive suppression of, in diagnosis of sick sinus syndrome, 140
as pacemaker of heart, 3-4
physiologic pause in discharge, as cause of interference-dissociation, 130-132
subnormal function; *see* Sick sinus syndrome
Sinus, carotid, stimulation of, in diagnosis of sick sinus syndrome, 140-141
Sinus arrhythmia, 14-15
Sinus bradycardia; *see* Bradycardia, sinus
Sinus rhythms, 13-15
conversion of atrial fibrillation to, 87-89
definition, 13
electrocardiographic diagnosis, 13
maintenance, 89
variations, 13-15
Sinus syndrome, sick; *see* Sick sinus syndrome
Sinus tachycardia, 13, 14
analysis, 169, 172-174
clinical differentiation from paroxysmal tachycardia, 34
Sodium bicarbonate for ventricular fibrillation, 153
Stokes-Adams seizures
in atrioventricular block, 78
due to atrioventricular block in bundle system, 71
as rationale for treatment of atrioventricular block, 80
Supraventricular beats, 18
Supraventricular paroxysmal tachycardia; *see* Paroxysmal tachycardia, supraventricular
Sustained ectopic rhythms; *see* Ectopic rhythms, sustained
Sympathetic nerve fibers, effects on conducting system, 6
Sympathomimetic drugs for supraventricular tachycardia, 35
Syncope
as symptom of atrioventricular block, 78
as symptom of sick sinus syndrome, 135

T

T waves
notching, in escape ectopic rhythms, 39-41
P waves buried in, in premature atrial beats, 21-22
vulnerable zone, 150
Tachycardia
atrial
and atrioventricular junctional, 31-33

Tachycardia—cont'd
atrial—cont'd
multifocal, 135
paroxysmal, edrophonium for, diagnosis, 182
junctional, induced by digitalis toxicity, 168-169
paroxysmal; *see* Paroxysmal tachycardia
sinus, 13, 14
analysis, 169, 172-174
clinical differentiation from paroxysmal tachycardia, 34
supraventricular, paroxysmal
beta-adrenergic blocking agents for, 183
edrophonium for, 182
ventricular; *see* Ventricular tachycardia
Tensilon; *see* Edrophonium
Thrombi, mural, in chronic atrial fibrillation, 84
Thyrotoxicosis as cause of atrial fibrillation, 82
Time measurements in electrocardiogram, 8-10
Transthoracic resistance to defibrillator current, reduction of, 190-191
Treatment
of atrial fibrillation, 87-90
of atrial flutter, 96-97
of atrioventricular block, 79-80
complete, 80
first-degree, 79
second-degree, 79
of digitalis-induced arrhythmias, 125-126
of escape or passive ectopic rhythms, 41-42
of fatal arrhythmia, 152-154
of interference-dissociation, 133-134
of paroxysmal tachycardia, 34-38
supraventricular, 35-36
ventricular, 36-38
of sick sinus syndrome, 141
of ventricular fibrillation, 152-153
of ventricular standstill, 153-154
Trifascicular block, 75-76

V

Vagal nerve fibers, effect on conducting system, 6
Vagal stimulation in paroxysmal tachycardia, 34
Vagomimetic drugs for supraventricular tachycardia, 35
Valium as premedication for cardioversion, 195
Ventricular beats, 19
Ventricular fibrillation; *see* Fibrillation, ventricular
Ventricular flutter, 150-152
Ventricular pacing, 187
in treatment of sick sinus syndrome, 141
in treatment of ventricular standstill, 153
Ventricular (QRS) complex
aberrations, 44-46
rate-dependent, analysis, 51
in atrioventricular block localized in bundle branches, 72-73, 74
in diagnosis of arrhythmias, 6
fusion, 46-49
irregular, in diagnosis of atrial fibrillation, 85
in isorhythmic dissociation, 133
narrow, in diagnosis of supraventricular paroxysmal tachycardia, 31
relation of P waves to, 20
widening, in diagnosis of pre-excitation, 160
Ventricular (QRS) interval in fascicular block, 75

Ventricular rate, slowing, 89-90
Ventricular rhythm, chaotic, 148
Ventricular standstill, 152
   treatment, 153-154
Ventricular tachycardia, 33-34, 36-38
   lidocaine for, 182
   multifocal, 148
   paroxysmal; *see* Paroxysmal tachycardia, ventricu-
      lar
   procainamide for, 181
   quinidine for, 180-181
   ventricular flutter following, 152
Vertigo
   as symptom of atrioventricular block, 78
   as symptom of sick sinus syndrome, 135

W

Wandering pacemaker, 158, 159
Waves of electrocardiogram
   correlation with, 4-6
   nomenclature, 8, 9
   P; *see* P waves
   T; *see* T waves
Wenckebach phenomenon, 62, 64-68
   analysis, 105-106, 109-110
   due to digitalis toxicity, 116, 118, 120
   localized in bundle branches, 73
Wolff-Parkinson-White syndrome, 158-161
   beta-adrenergic blocking agents for, 183

X

Xylocaine for ventricular tachycardia, 36-37